306.1   B
AUG   August

Druds & Women

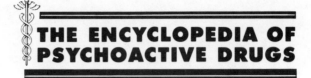

THE ENCYCLOPEDIA OF PSYCHOACTIVE DRUGS

SERIES 1

Alcohol And Alcoholism
Alcohol Customs & Rituals
Alcohol Teenage Drinking
Flowering Plants Magic in Bloom
LSD Visions or Nightmares
Marijuana Its Effects on Mind & Body
Mushrooms Psychedelic Fungi
PCP The Dangerous Angel
Heroin The Street Narcotic
Methadone Treatment for Addiction
Prescription Narcotics The Addictive Painkillers
Over-the-Counter Drugs Harmless or Hazardous?
Barbiturates Sleeping Potion or Intoxicant?

Inhalants The Toxic Fumes
Quaaludes The Quest for Oblivion
Valium The Tranquil Trap
Amphetamines Danger in the Fast Lane
Caffeine The Most Popular Stimulant
Cocaine A New Epidemic
Nicotine An Old-Fashioned Addiction
The Addictive Personality
Escape from Anxiety and Stress
Getting Help Treatments for Drug Abuse
Treating Mental Illness
Teenage Depression and Drugs

SERIES 2

Bad Trips
Brain Function
Case Histories
Celebrity Drug Use
Designer Drugs
Drinking, Driving, and Drugs
The Down Side of Drugs
Drugs and Crime
Drugs and Diet
Drugs and Disease
Drugs and Emotion
Drugs and Pain
Drugs and Perception
Drugs and Pregnancy
Drugs and Sexual Behavior
Drugs and Sleep

Drugs and Sports
Drugs and the Arts
Drugs and the Brain
Drugs and the Family
Drugs and the Law
Drugs and Women
Drugs in Civilization
Drugs of the Future
Drugs Through the Ages
Drug Use Around the World
Legalization A Debate
Mental Disturbances
Nutrition and the Brain
The Origins and Sources of Drugs
Substance Abuse Prevention and Cures
Who Uses Drugs?

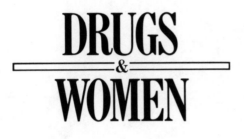

DRUGS
& WOMEN

GENERAL EDITOR
Professor Solomon H. Snyder, M.D.

*Distinguished Service Professor of
Neuroscience, Pharmacology, and Psychiatry at
The Johns Hopkins University School of Medicine*

•

ASSOCIATE EDITOR
Professor Barry L. Jacobs, Ph.D.

*Program in Neuroscience, Department of Psychology,
Princeton University*

•

SENIOR EDITORIAL CONSULTANT
Joann Rodgers

*Deputy Director, Office of Public Affairs at
The Johns Hopkins Medical Institutions*

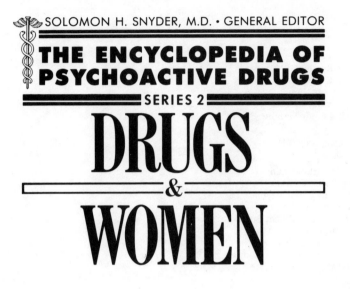

SOLOMON H. SNYDER, M.D. • GENERAL EDITOR

THE ENCYCLOPEDIA OF PSYCHOACTIVE DRUGS

SERIES 2

DRUGS
&
WOMEN

PAUL NORDSTROM AUGUST

CHELSEA HOUSE PUBLISHERS
NEW YORK • NEW HAVEN • PHILADELPHIA

EDITOR-IN-CHIEF: Nancy Toff
EXECUTIVE EDITOR: Remmel T. Nunn
MANAGING EDITOR: Karyn Gullen Browne
COPY CHIEF: Perry Scott King
ART DIRECTOR: Giannella Garrett
PICTURE EDITOR: Elizabeth Terhune

Staff for DRUGS AND WOMEN:

SENIOR EDITOR: Jane Larkin Crain
ASSOCIATE EDITOR: Paula Edelson
ASSISTANT EDITOR: Michele A. Merens
DESIGNER: Victoria Tomaselli
COPY EDITORS: Sean Dolan, Gillian Bucky
CAPTIONS: Louise Bloomfield
PICTURE RESEARCH: Emily Miller
PRODUCTION COORDINATOR: Alma Rodriguez
PRODUCTION ASSISTANT: Karen Dreste

CREATIVE DIRECTOR: Harold Steinberg

COVER: Giorgio de Chirico, *The Soothsayer's Recompense,* Philadelphia Museum
of Art: The Louise and Walter Arensberg Collection

Library of Congress Cataloging-in-Publication Data
August, Paul
  Drugs & women
  (Encyclopedia of psychoactive drugs. Series 2)
  Bibliography: p.
  Includes index.
  Summary: Examines the increasing use and effects
of drugs, both legal and illicit, among women in
today's society and the sociological and cultural
reasons for this phenomenon.
    1. Substance abuse—Juvenile literature. 2.
Women—Substance use—Juvenile literature. [1. Drug
abuse. 2. Women—Drug abuse. 3. Drugs] I. Title. II.
Title: Drugs and women. III. Series. [1. Substance
Abuse—popular works. 2. Women—popular works.
WM 270 A923]
RC564.A92   1987   306'.1   86-34346

ISBN 1-55546-227-8

CONTENTS

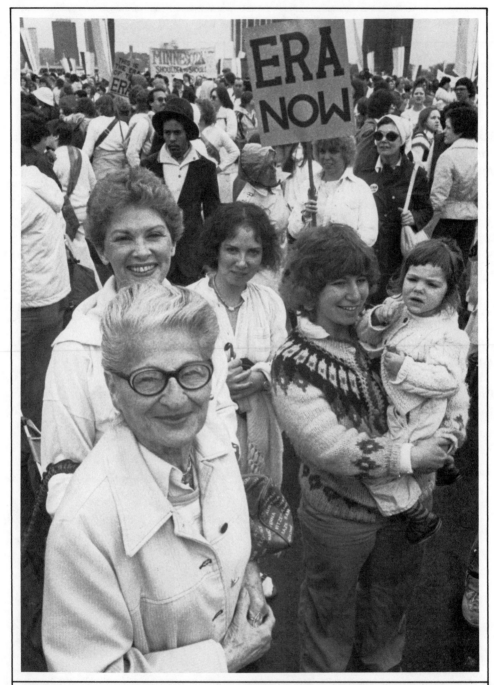

Four generations of women demonstrate in favor of the Equal Rights Amendment. Women have greater opportunities in the 1980s than ever before but are also forced to deal with new stresses and conflicts.

FOREWORD

In the Mainstream
of American Life

One of the legacies of the social upheaval of the 1960s is that psychoactive drugs have become part of the mainstream of American life. Schools, homes, and communities cannot be "drug proofed." There is a demand for drugs — and the supply is plentiful. Social norms have changed and drugs are not only available—they are everywhere.

But where efforts to curtail the supply of drugs and outlaw their use have had tragically limited effects on demand, it may be that education has begun to stem the rising tide of drug abuse among young people and adults alike.

Over the past 25 years, as drugs have become an increasingly routine facet of contemporary life, a great many teenagers have adopted the notion that drug taking was somehow a right or a privilege or a necessity. They have done so, however, without understanding the consequences of drug use during the crucial years of adolescence.

The teenage years are few in the total life cycle, but critical in the maturation process. During these years adolescents face the difficult tasks of discovering their identity, clarifying their sexual roles, asserting their independence, learning to cope with authority, and searching for goals that will give their lives meaning.

Drugs rob adolescents of precious time, stamina, and health. They interrupt critical learning processes, sometimes forever. Teenagers who use drugs are likely to withdraw increasingly into themselves, to "cop out" at just the time when they most need to reach out and experience the world.

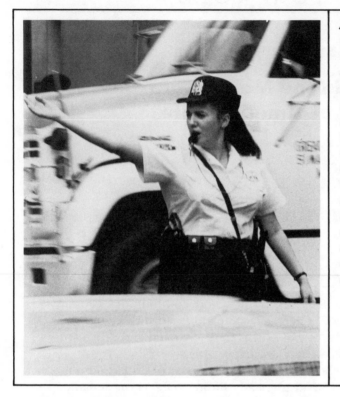

A policewoman directs traffic in New York City. Full-time employment is becoming a norm for both single and married women. As the demands placed on them at work and at home become more various and complex, some women turn to alcohol and other drugs in a self-defeating attempt to cope with anxiety and tension.

Fortunately, as a recent Gallup poll shows, young people are beginning to realize this, too. They themselves label drugs their most important problem. In the last few years, moreover, the climate of tolerance and ignorance surrounding drugs has been changing.

Adolescents as well as adults are becoming aware of mounting evidence that every race, ethnic group, and class is vulnerable to drug dependency.

Recent publicity about the cost and failure of drug rehabilitation efforts; dangerous drug use among pilots, air traffic controllers, star athletes, and Hollywood celebrities; and drug-related accidents, suicides, and violent crime have focused the public's attention on the need to wage an all-out war on drug abuse before it seriously undermines the fabric of society itself.

The anti-drug message is getting stronger and there is evidence that the message is beginning to get through to adults and teenagers alike.

The Encyclopedia of Psychoactive Drugs hopes to play a part in the national campaign now underway to educate young people about drugs. Series 1 provides clear and comprehensive discussions of common psychoactive substances, outlines their psychological and physiological effects on the mind and body, explains how they "hook" the user, and separates fact from myth in the complex issue of drug abuse.

Whereas Series 1 focuses on specific drugs, such as nicotine or cocaine, Series 2 confronts a broad range of both social and physiological phenomena. Each volume addresses the ramifications of drug use and abuse on some aspect of human experience: social, familial, cultural, historical, and physical. Separate volumes explore questions about the effects of drugs on brain chemistry and unborn children; the use and abuse of painkillers; the relationship between drugs and sexual behavior, sports, and the arts; drugs and disease; the role of drugs in history and the sophisticated drugs now being developed in the laboratory that will profoundly change the future.

Each book in the series is fully illustrated and is tailored to the needs and interests of young readers. The more adolescents know about drugs and their role in society, the less likely they are to misuse them.

Joann Rodgers
Senior Editorial Consultant

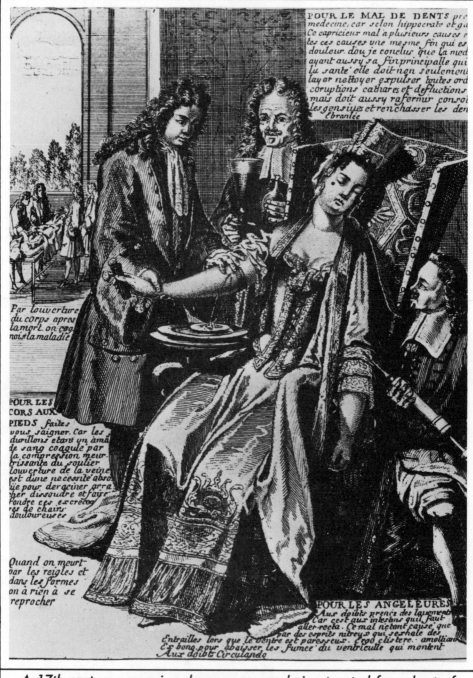

POUR LE MAL DE DENTS pre
medecine, car selon hippocrate et ga
Ce capricieux mal a plusieurs causes e
les ces causes une mesme fin qui es
douleur, dou je conclus que la med
ayant aussy sa fin principalle qui
lu sante' elle doit non seulement
lay er nettoyer expulser toutes ord
coruptions cathares et defluctions
mais doit aussy rafermir consoi
les gensiues et renchasser les den
Ebranlée

Par l'ouverture
du corps apres
la mort, on con
noist la maladie

POUR LES
CORS AUX
PIEDS faites
vous saigner. Car les
durillons etant un ama
de sang coagule par
la compression meur
trissante du soulier
l'ouverture de la veine
est d'une necessité abso
lije pour deraciner arra
her dissoudre et faire
fondre ces excrecoi
res de chairs
douloureuses

Quand on meurt
par les reigles et
dans les formes
on a rien a se
reprocher

POUR LES ANGELEURES
Aux doibts prenez des lavements
Car c'est aux interins qu'il faut
aller rocha. Ce mal netant cause que
par des esprits nitreux qui sexhale des
Entrailles lors que le ventre est paresseux. Ergo clistere. amollian
Et bon pour abaisser les fumée du ventricule qui montent
Aux doibts Circulande

A 17th-century engraving shows a woman being treated for a host of ailments. Statistics show that women in contemporary society turn to doctors and prescription drugs more frequently than do men.

INTRODUCTION

The Gift of Wizardry
Use and Abuse

JACK H. MENDELSON, M.D.
NANCY K. MELLO, PH.D.

Alcohol and Drug Abuse Research Center
Harvard Medical School—McLean Hospital

Dorothy to the Wizard:

"I think you are a very bad man," said Dorothy.
"Oh no, my dear; I'm really a very good man; but I'm a very bad Wizard."

—from THE WIZARD OF OZ

Man is endowed with the gift of wizardry, a talent for discovery and invention. The discovery and invention of substances that change the way we feel and behave are among man's special accomplishments, and, like so many other products of our wizardry, these substances have the capacity to harm as well as to help. Psychoactive drugs can cause profound changes in the chemistry of the brain and other vital organs, and although their legitimate use can relieve pain and cure disease, their abuse leads in a tragic number of cases to destruction.

Consider alcohol — available to all and yet regarded with intense ambivalence from biblical times to the present day. The use of alcoholic beverages dates back to our earliest ancestors. Alcohol use and misuse became associated with the worship of gods and demons. One of the most powerful Greek gods was Dionysus, lord of fruitfulness and god of wine. The Romans adopted Dionysus but changed his name to Bacchus. Festivals and holidays associated with Bacchus celebrated the harvest and the origins of life. Time has blurred the images of the Bacchanalian festival, but the theme of drunkenness as a major part of celebration has survived the pagan gods and remains a familiar part of modern society. The term "Bacchanalian Festival" conveys a more appealing image than "drunken orgy" or "pot party," but whatever the label, drinking alcohol is a form of drug use that results in addiction for millions.

The fact that many millions of other people can use alcohol in moderation does not mitigate the toll this drug takes on society as a whole. According to reliable estimates, one out of every ten Americans develops a serious alcohol-related problem sometime in his or her lifetime. In addition, automobile accidents caused by drunken drivers claim the lives of tens of thousands every year. Many of the victims are gifted young people, just starting out in adult life. Hospital emergency rooms abound with patients seeking help for al-cohol-related injuries.

Who is to blame? Can we blame the many manufacturers who produce such an amazing variety of alcoholic beverages? Should we blame the educators who fail to explain the perils of intoxication, or so exaggerate the dangers of drinking that no one could possibly believe them? Are friends to blame — those peers who urge others to "drink more and faster," or the macho types who stress the importance of being able to "hold your liquor"? Casting blame, however, is hardly con-structive, and pointing the finger is a fruitless way to deal with the problem. Alcoholism and drug abuse have few cul-prits but many victims. Accountability begins with each of us, every time we choose to use or misuse an intoxicating substance.

It is ironic that some of man's earliest medicines, derived from natural plant products, are used today to poison and to intoxicate. Relief from pain and suffering is one of society's many continuing goals. Over 3,000 years ago, the Therapeutic Papyrus of Thebes, one of our earliest written records, gave instructions for the use of opium in the treatment of pain. Opium, in the form of its major derivative, morphine, and similar compounds, such as heroin, have also been used by many to induce changes in mood and feeling. Another ex-ample of man's misuse of a natural substance is the coca leaf, which for centuries was used by the Indians of Peru to reduce fatigue and hunger. Its modern derivative, cocaine, has im-portant medical use as a local anesthetic. Unfortunately, its increasing abuse in the 1980s clearly has reached epidemic proportions.

The purpose of this series is to explore in depth the psychological and behavioral effects that psychoactive drugs have on the individual, and also, to investigate the ways in which drug use influences the legal, economic, cultural, and even moral aspects of societies. The information presented here (and in other books in this series) is based on many clinical and laboratory studies and other observations by people from diverse walks of life.

Over the centuries, novelists, poets, and dramatists have provided us with many insights into the sometimes seductive but ultimately problematic aspects of alcohol and drug use. Physicians, lawyers, biologists, psychologists, and social scientists have contributed to a better understanding of the causes and consequences of using these substances. The authors in this series have attempted to gather and condense all the latest information about drug use and abuse. They have also described the sometimes wide gaps in our knowledge and have suggested some new ways to answer many difficult questions.

One such question, for example, is how do alcohol and drug problems get started? And what is the best way to treat them when they do? Not too many years ago, alcoholics and drug abusers were regarded as evil, immoral, or both. It is now recognized that these persons suffer from very complicated diseases involving deep psychological and social problems. To understand how the disease begins and progresses, it is necessary to understand the nature of the substance, the behavior of addicts, and the characteristics of the society or culture in which they live.

Although many of the social environments we live in are very similar, some of the most subtle differences can strongly influence our thinking and behavior. Where we live, go to school and work, whom we discuss things with — all influence our opinions about drug use and misuse. Yet we also share certain commonly accepted beliefs that outweigh any differences in our attitudes. The authors in this series have tried to identify and discuss the central, most crucial issues concerning drug use and misuse.

Despite the increasing sophistication of the chemical substances we create in the laboratory, we have a long way to go in our efforts to make these powerful drugs work for us rather than against us.

The volumes in this series address a wide range of timely questions. What influence has drug use had on the arts? Why do so many of today's celebrities and star athletes use drugs, and what is being done to solve this problem? What is the relationship between drugs and crime? What is the physiological basis for the power drugs can hold over us? These are but a few of the issues explored in this far-ranging series.

Educating people about the dangers of drugs can go a long way towards minimizing the desperate consequences of substance abuse for individuals and society as a whole. Luckily, human beings have the resources to solve even the most serious problems that beset them, once they make the commitment to do so. As one keen and sensitive observer, Dr. Lewis Thomas, has said,

> There is nothing at all absurd about the human condition. We matter. It seems to me a good guess, hazarded by a good many people who have thought about it, that we may be engaged in the formation of something like a mind for the life of this planet. If this is so, we are still at the most primitive stage, still fumbling with language and thinking, but infinitely capacitated for the future. Looked at this way, it is remarkable that we've come as far as we have in so short a period, really no time at all as geologists measure time. We are the newest, youngest, and the brightest thing around.

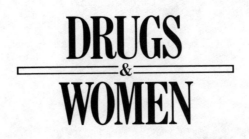

DRUGS
& WOMEN

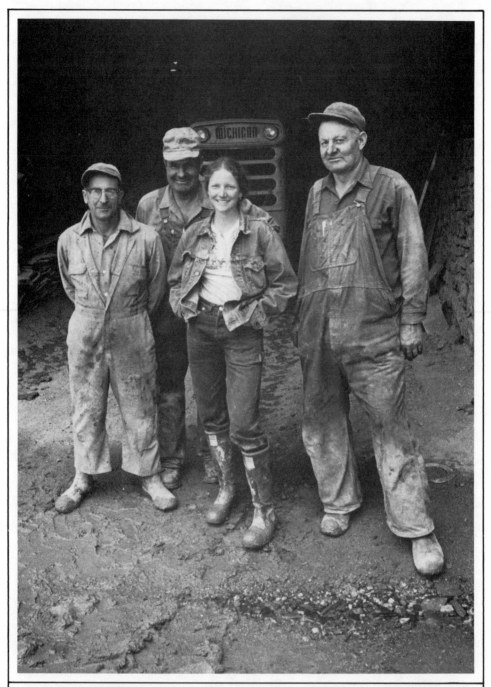

A 17-year-old miner poses with three of her colleagues. Women who hold full-time jobs often must work harder than their male peers to succeed in what has traditionally been a "man's world."

AUTHOR'S PREFACE

In one sense, it might be argued, a book on women and drugs is unnecessary. At a certain level of consideration — and by no means an unsophisticated one — the many effects of human drug use are independent of gender. Recent research by molecular biologists, psychopharmacologists, and other scientists has clarified the modes of action of many common drugs — such as heroin, Valium, tobacco, and cocaine — at the cellular level. For the most part, psychoactive drugs affect the user's mood by somehow modifying, blocking, or mimicking the natural actions of the body's *neurotransmitters*. These are the chemicals involved in the transmission of information within the tremendously complicated network of neurons (or nerve cells) that makes up the human brain.

Scientists have discovered that heroin and other opiates exert their variety of effects by acting on natural opiate receptors throughout the body. Cocaine, for example, prevents the neurotransmitter norepinephrine from reentering the neuron from which it was released, thereby increasing the effects of this neurotransmitter. Antianxiety pills such as Valium work by increasing the effects of an inhibitory neurotransmitter, *gamma-aminobutyric acid* (GABA), at natural GABA receptors. The effects of these drugs are essentially the same, at this level, in both men and women.

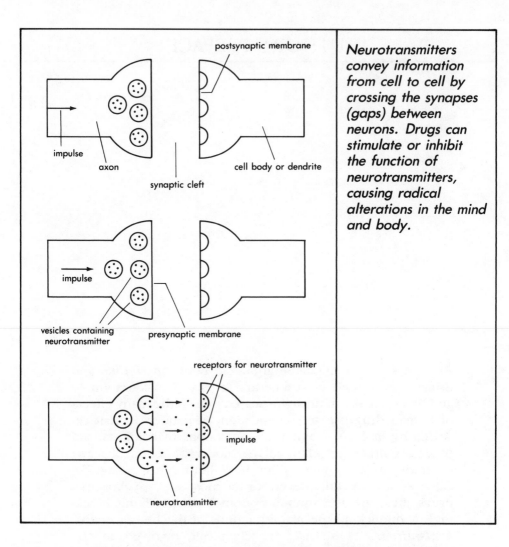

Neurotransmitters convey information from cell to cell by crossing the synapses (gaps) between neurons. Drugs can stimulate or inhibit the function of neurotransmitters, causing radical alterations in the mind and body.

There are, however, certain biological differences between men and women that lead to distinct responses to various drugs, especially with regard to physiological side effects. This is obviously of vital importance with regard to female reproductive biology. Whereas the primary reproductive role of the man involves only the relatively simple process of *spermatogenesis* (sperm formation) and eventual fertilization of the woman during intercourse, the role of the woman is much more complex and can have a much greater impact on the health of the offspring. The woman not only produces an ovum but also nourishes and protects the fetus during gestation; additionally, in most cases she cares for the child after birth. A variety of drugs taken before, during, and after pregnancy can adversely affect the health of both the mother and the child.

Even women who do not immediately intend to bear children can suffer from the side effects of some drugs. Some substances can disrupt the menstrual cycle in certain ways. Others can decrease the effectiveness or increase the hazards of the oral contraceptive (birth control) pill. This is of special significance to many modern women, who may be more sexually active than women of previous generations, and who may also often find themselves, and not their male partners, responsible for any contraceptive precautions taken.

Additionally, when the reasons for taking psychoactive drugs are considered, it becomes clear that the use of virtually any drug can be related to specific trends involving women and cause special problems for them. Human psychology cannot easily be divorced from sociology; women's social roles, which are undergoing dramatic changes, create distinct patterns, circumstances, and consequences of drug use. This is especially significant because many drugs — alcohol and tranquilizers are two obvious examples — are used in response to stressful life situations. Many women in Western society today — be they full-time homemakers, career-minded professionals, single mothers, or married women trying to juggle both career and family — lead lives characterized by tension and a lack of personal time. Factors such as these are at least partially responsible for the fact that use of several drugs by women is increasing, while use of the same substances by men has leveled off or is even decreasing.

This book investigates physiological, psychological, and sociological aspects of drug use by women. Chapter 1 discusses some of the causes and overall patterns of substance abuse and also the consequences of that abuse. Chapters 2 through 7 are devoted to reviews of drug families — alcohol, tobacco, tranquilizers, stimulants, opiates, and marijuana — and the specific ways they can affect women. Chapter 8 describes the most important effects of the use of several psychoactive drugs during pregnancy. Finally, Chapter 9 considers the special position of teenage women and actions of the drugs to which they are most likely to be exposed.

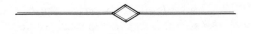

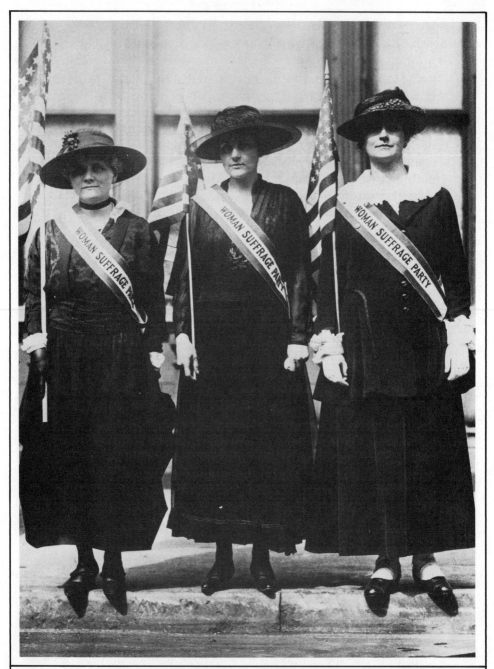

Women throughout the United States campaigned for the right to vote in the early 20th century and won their battle when women's suffrage became law in 1920. The struggle for women's rights has continued to the present day in both the social and professional worlds.

CHAPTER 1

SOCIAL AND CULTURAL FACTORS

Over the last few decades the dramatic changes in the prevalence of drug use and the ever-expanding variety of substances being used have been paralleled by enormous changes in the social roles and status of women and in the range of opportunities open to them. Although it would be foolhardy to propose a direct cause-and-effect relationship between these two trends, it is clear that changes in the patterns of drug use by women both reflect changing social and cultural trends and cause further such changes.

Perhaps most important have been the recent changes in family structure. Women of all ages obviously play one or more key roles in every family — most significantly, of course, as mother — and women are most likely to feel the full effects of changes in the family and in the "institution" of marriage. The enormous rise in the divorce rate and in the number of children born to unwed mothers (accounting for more than 50% of all births in some cities) has contributed to a virtual epidemic of one-parent families — and the single parent is usually the mother. For a variety of reasons, women from all sorts of educational and social backgrounds are present in the work force in unprecedented numbers. In fact, the traditional structure, in which the father works and the "housewife"-mother stays home with the children, now exists in less than a third of all American households.

How these and other social and cultural trends influence drug use by women are investigated in this chapter. It is sometimes difficult to label such factors as direct "causes" of drug use. Often it is more a question of interactions between factor and use. For example, family or occupational problems may precede alcohol abuse, which in turn exacerbates the original problems. Cocaine or heroin users may turn to prostitution out of economic necessity; on the other hand, the physical and emotional degradation associated with prostitution may perpetuate drug use. Even when the cause of drug use cannot be established, however, an awareness of these problems, forces, and pressures is crucial to an understanding of female drug use.

Teenagers and Changing Values

In many ways, teenagers today — and especially women — must bear the brunt of the confusion spawned by the changes in social values that have swept America since the late 1960s and early 1970s. In the last 25 or so years, traditional morality — with regard to both sexual behavior and drug use — has been profoundly altered. Today's high-school students, many of whom routinely engage in sexual activity and casual drug use, especially of marijuana, are in a sense victims of a social order that has discarded one set of norms without replacing it with anything else. In addition, the "flower children" of the 1960s now have children of their own, which has led to a situation in which teenagers may have parents who not only drink and smoke tobacco but also use marijuana, cocaine, or other illicit drugs.

The media and the entertainment industry have played an unfortunate role in determining the way teenagers regard drug use. On television, conflicting images of drug use appear: whereas network television generally portrays drug use in a negative light, the "home video revolution," involving cable networks and videocassette recorders, has introduced into the home more positive images of drug use. Many films of the 1970s and 1980s, particularly those aimed at young audiences, portray illicit drug use (generally of marijuana and cocaine) in glamorous or humorous ways. Contemporary music and musical personalities, now commonly seen on television music video shows, are also frequently associated with drug use. Similarly, alcohol use by teenagers is commonly

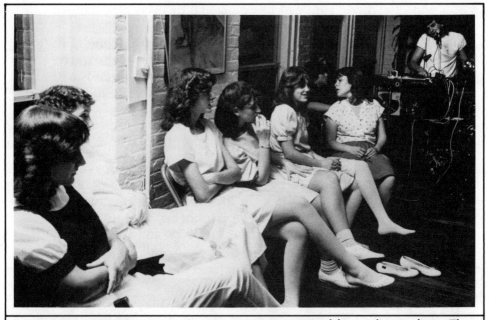

Guests at a "sweet sixteen" party are entertained by a disc jockey. The combination of peer pressure and the desire to be accepted has pushed many teenagers into experimenting with various drugs.

projected as fun, sophisticated, or humorous; although characters may occasionally get sick from their drinking, the long-term and decidedly unfunny and unsophisticated aspects of alcoholism are rarely seen.

Whatever the decade under consideration, the teenage years have always been a time of transition, stress, choices, and excitement. Many high-school students — young women more than ever before — hope to go on to higher education, and there is tremendous pressure to perform well academically. At the same time, complicating the struggle for good grades, various forms of social life beckon. Despite the many benefits of high-school social relationships, there are added problems and possible crises. To name but a few: rejection by a particular social group or member of the opposite sex; concerns with physical attractiveness and related issues such as weight; and sexual problems, including, most catastrophically, unwanted pregnancy. All these academic and social pressures, as well as the inevitable peer pressure at parties and elsewhere, can lead to occasional or even habitual use of drugs.

Teenage use of the most common drugs, alcohol and tobacco, is not new but is generally more frequent today, especially among teenage women. These modern trends will be discussed in later chapters devoted specifically to these substances.

Women and Families

Many people use drugs not for recreational purposes but as an escape from stress, depression, or other types of emotional turmoil. Rather than work on long-term solutions to their problems, some women turn to alcohol and tranquilizers as a means of coping with marital troubles and the ongoing

Just as women have become a vital part of the work force, they have also had to face the emotional stress of unemployment. This can be overwhelming, especially when a woman has a child to support. Psychoactive drugs, frequently prescribed by doctors, offer temporary relief, but long-term solutions must include economic and social reforms.

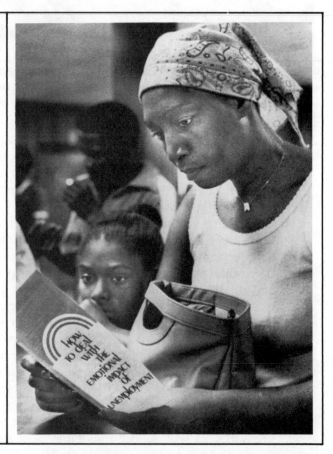

tribulations of motherhood. In this they are abetted by a medical establishment that too often dismisses female complaints with a prescription for Valium when counseling and support are what is really needed. (This aspect of drug dependence is discussed later in this chapter.)

Raising children has of course never been easy, but in contemporary society it can be especially difficult. Many young mothers are separated, divorced, or unwed and thus must handle the strains of part-time or full-time work in addition to caring for their children. Periods of unemployment (and the resulting poverty) can be especially traumatic for these women. Angry and unhappy relations with former husbands or boyfriends can readily cause further emotional strain.

Even for women with outwardly stable marriages, life in the 1980s is full of stressful challenges. Suburban life can seem lonely, sterile, and lacking in social cohesiveness. Frequently the husband must spend a great deal of time commuting to his job, with the result that he sees little of his wife and family. After suffering the inevitable pressures of an urban job and commute, he returns home full of his own frustrations. The children's schooling (generally the responsibility of the mother) may be the cause of a variety of problems, not least of which may be adolescent sexual activity or drug use.

Occupational Hazards

As noted, more women are now working outside the home than ever before. In some instances, this is largely by choice or by intention: female college graduates are just as likely to be interested in a long-term professional career as their male classmates; older married women may seek an interesting job once their children have grown up and they are freed from the limitations of mothering. In other cases it is due more to simple economic necessity — the single mother, the wife forced to work to supplement family income, or the young woman who turns to prostitution to maintain an expensive drug habit such as heroin addiction.

Whatever the motivation for working and whatever the nature of the job — from traditional female occupations such as secretarial work, modeling, waitressing, and nursing to more "liberated," professional work in business, law, medi-

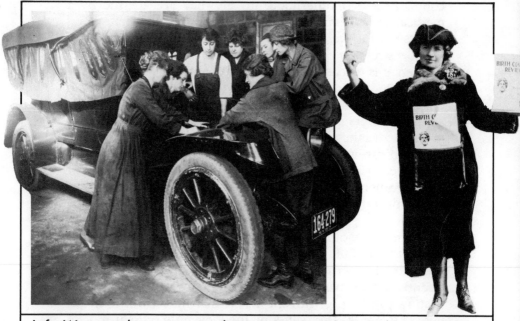

Left: Women take an auto mechanics course in 1917. Right: Activist Kitty Marion sells copies of the Birth Control Review in 1916. Both activities are examples of early strides towards women's rights.

cine, and politics — it is certain that women face stresses and difficulties different from those encountered by men. Despite some feminist success in the area of equal rights in the workplace, in many if not most jobs (save for traditional "feminine" ones) it is still harder for a woman to be hired and promoted, and her wages tend to be less than those of her male counterparts.

Working women must often deal with other pressures. For instance, many women must balance perceived needs to look and act "feminine" in the office and at home while at the same time acting as competitively and as "macho" as their male colleagues. Similar confusion may also exist as to how far a woman can and should join in traditional, previously all-male social aspects of work, typified by after-work drinking sessions or weekend golf with business associates. There are obvious further complications with such work-related socializing, whether the woman is married or single.

Sexual harassment, both subtle and overt, in the office and at the bar after work, is a clear and common problem faced by women in almost any line of work — from secretaries and nurses up to those in the highest echelons of business. Often, being hired or promoted is linked, at times even explicitly, with acquiescence to an employer's sexual demands. Even in the absence of such direct propositions and threats, women can be the target of sexist comments and sexual innuendo. Anger, bitterness, resentment, feelings of powerlessness, and fears for one's job are the obvious, understandable results of such chauvinism and harassment.

Other work-related problems can exist. In the common two-career household where both parents work, it tends to fall upon the mother to care for the children and manage the household chores rather than upon the father, even if they work equal hours. Additional occupational complications can arise during pregnancy. Marital problems can also be aggravated by a wife's career, often when a husband is uncomfortable with her decision to work. He may have traditional attitudes involving a wife's staying at home, feelings of guilt or insecurity if his lack of a job or insufficient income has

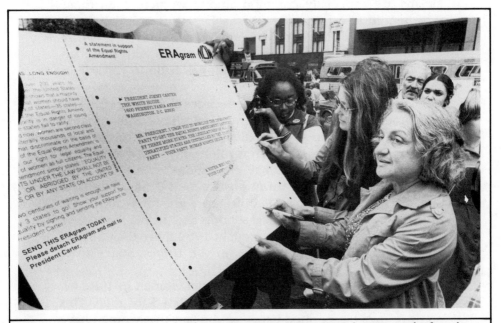

Betty Friedan (front) and Gloria Steinem campaigned vigorously for the Equal Rights Amendment. The ERA, which was not ratified, was meant to secure such liberties for women as "equal pay for equal work."

forced his wife to work, or he may be threatened by her autonomy.

Thus, despite progress toward equality in the workplace, women working outside the home continue to encounter discrimination, prejudice, harassment, and confusion with regard to what has been termed their "dual-sex roles" — as well as the normal stresses and pressures inherent in any job, whether held by male or female. Once again, with reference to female drug use such occupational hazards influence not so much recreational or social use (although some job-related drug problems undoubtedly start as such) but rather the abuse of drugs as a means to cope with anxiety and tension. Needless to say, such coping behavior by means of drugs is not unique to women; alcoholism among men has often been linked to career stress.

Women and the Medical Establishment

Problems with legal psychoactive drugs such as the tranquilizers and stimulants prescribed by psychiatrists and physicians are especially common among women, even those who would never consider themselves drug abusers or addicts of any kind. Part of this phenomenon is due to the nature of the medical establishment, its relationship with the pharmaceutical industry, and its traditional attitude toward its female patients.

Although certainly in recent decades increasing numbers of women have been entering medical school and going on to practice in all areas of medicine, the overall medical establishment — and particularly its hierarchy — is overwhelmingly male. With occasional exceptions, most heads of professional medical organizations are men, deans of medical schools and their admissions directors are men, and those who teach students in medical schools and hospitals are men. Moreover, most doctors are men: in 1982 more than 85% of the roughly 500,000 physicians in the United States were male.

Most patients, however, are female: women in 1982 averaged 5.8 visits per year compared with 4.5 for men. This statistic may be ascribed partly to the fact that women have traditionally been less expected than men to bear emotional problems such as depression and anxiety in silence and are therefore more likely to visit their doctor for assistance. This

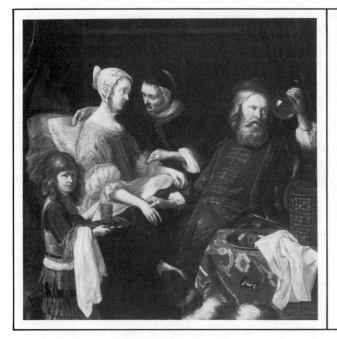

The Sick Woman, *by Jacob Toorenvliet. Although the traditional stereotype of women as delicate, disease-prone creatures is outmoded, many contemporary male doctors persist in the belief that more women than men need prescription drugs to help them deal with psychological and physical ailments.*

may represent a change from earlier eras, when a religious figure, such as a priest or rabbi, might have handled these problems.

Unlike their religious counterparts, however, doctors and psychiatrists often rely on psychoactive drugs to "cure" their female patients of a variety of emotional problems such as anxiety, insomnia (sleeplessness), depression, or simple recurring pains. Unfortunately this pharmaceutical approach tends to cure the symptoms but does not address the problems behind them. For example, sleeping pills may help resolve insomnia but will not cure the anxiety or depression causing it.

There are several reasons why this "prescription pad" approach prevails. Traditional medical education places a tremendous emphasis on pharmacological remedies for virtually all conditions, particularly psychological problems such as depression or anxiety. This educational bias toward drug treatment is further bolstered by continuous pressure from the pharmaceutical companies that manufacture and market these drugs. The pharmaceutical industry is also one of the major advertisers in most of the leading medical journals, as well as the publisher of free newsletters of their own, which are sent automatically to doctors. Partly as a result of such intensive promotional techniques, the tranquilizer Valium was for many years the most commonly prescribed drug in the United States. (Reflecting increased fears about its side effects and addictive potential, its sales slipped slightly during the late 1970s and early 1980s.)

There are other reasons why doctors are quick to prescribe psychoactive drugs for their patients. In part this is due to cultural attitudes toward sickness. Problems — especially psychological ones — formerly treated by discussion, compassion, rest, common sense, or other methods are now almost automatically treated by "wonder drugs" of one sort or another, at times despite hazardous side effects or potential addiction.

As mentioned earlier, women are generally considered less able to bear pain than men — either physical or psychological — and male doctors often assume a paternalistic attitude toward their female patients. In addition, many doctors believe that patients would feel "cheated" if they left the

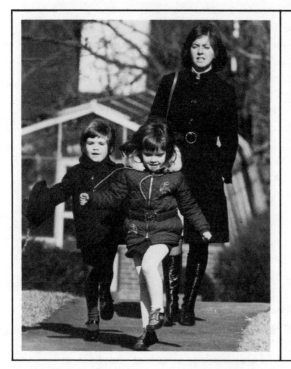

Working women with children cite child care as the greatest problem they face in juggling job and family obligations. Here, a woman cares for a friend's children and her own on her appointed day to watch both sets of youngsters.

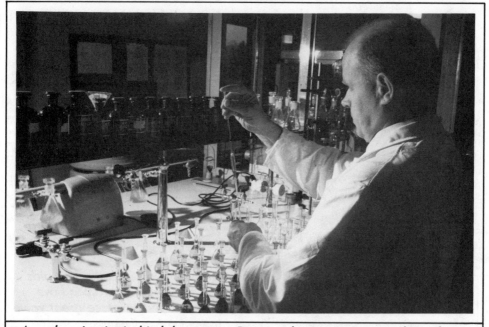

A male scientist in his laboratory. Despite the increasing number of women enrolled in medical schools, most doctors in the 1980s are male.

office without some sort of prescription in their hands. Others say that the patient will get the drug somehow in any case, so it might as well be from them.

General Cultural Attitudes Toward Women

In addition to the fairly well defined influences discussed above, pervasive cultural stereotypes and attitudes can play roles in encouraging drug use in certain women. From a very early age, girls learn the importance and value of physical attractiveness — in getting attention from boys, succeeding in job interviews, and finding mates. This cultural value, which is often exhibited and reinforced by magazine articles, films, and television, can have several effects upon drug use by women. In a general sense, women with low self-esteem may turn to drugs out of frustration or as an escape. More specifically, women with weight problems may abuse amphetamines in the hope that these stimulants will help them lose weight. Similarly, some women will not give up

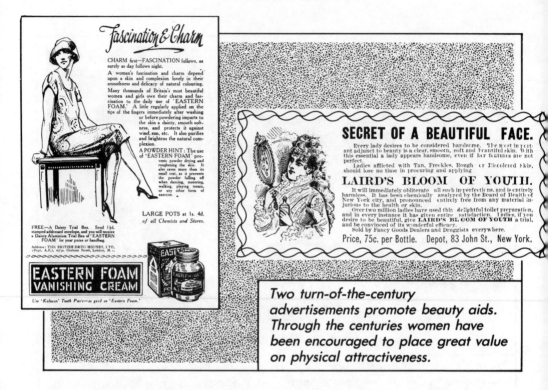

Two turn-of-the-century advertisements promote beauty aids. Through the centuries women have been encouraged to place great value on physical attractiveness.

cigarette smoking because they are afraid they will gain weight.

There are other examples of how such cultural sexism can lead to potential drug problems. Some women worry about aging, partly as a result of the premium society places on youth and attractiveness in women. An older single woman may find it harder to marry or to form intimate relationships than a man her age would. This has clear importance inasmuch as loneliness, feelings of being discarded, and related depression are important common precursors of drug abuse by women, especially alcoholism.

The effects of drug abuse in men and women are also subject to different interpretations according to gender. One common example concerns alcohol: a man who is drunk may be treated humorously, as "one of the boys," or even in some situations with a certain amount of respect, whereas an inebriated woman is often scorned or insulted and sometimes taken advantage of sexually. Partly as a result of such chauvinism, women sometimes hide their drinking or use of other substances as much as possible — in some cases thus further aggravating their drug problems.

In recent years much has been done to eliminate discrimination against women and to change unfair and sexist cultural attitudes toward them. Clearly, however, women in the 1980s continue to face difficult times both in the home and in the workplace. The various pressures created by the difficult roles imposed on women are clearly related to recent increases in some types of drug use by women. In addition, changing social mores and increasing permissiveness have led to new, relaxed attitudes toward recreational drug use, particularly during high-school and college years. The following chapters examine what some of these drugs can do to a woman's mind and body.

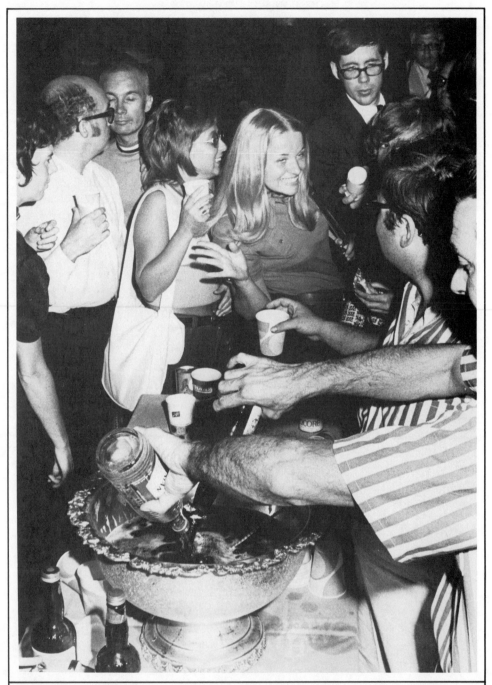

Social drinking is an accepted custom among adults of both sexes, but alcoholism, which is sometimes the next step, is a devastating disease that is afflicting an increasing amount of women as well as men.

CHAPTER 2

WOMEN AND ALCOHOL

Despite the clear hazards associated with the use of a variety of illicit drugs, abuse of the legal substance alcohol remains, along with the use of tobacco, America's greatest drug problem. Alcohol's legal status ensures easy availability, low prices relative to other drugs, social acceptance, and billion-dollar advertising campaigns aimed at promoting alcohol consumption. Drinking is portrayed constantly and often glamorously in books, films, and television series. All these factors combine to create an enormous alcohol problem among virtually all classes, races, and nationalities. Some recent evidence suggests that drinking among teenagers has risen over the last few decades; women of all ages are also using alcohol more. Alcohol's effects on women and the problems associated with alcohol abuse by women are the subject of this chapter.

General Features of Alcohol

Alcohol, more technically termed *ethanol* or *ethyl alcohol*, is a small chemical substance that readily travels in the bloodstream to enter virtually every area of the body. Its effects on the brain and other vital organs such as the heart and liver are complex and widespread, but they may be easily summarized: although its use is socially accepted, alcohol is a poison. The harmful aspects of drinking can be loosely divided into acute effects, which occur immediately after heavy or "binge" drinking, and chronic effects, which result from long-term alcohol abuse.

Acute Effects

Ethanol is classified as a *central nervous system depressant*, which means that it acts to depress or lower the brain's functions, as do barbiturates, Valium, and other "downers." The liveliness, good humor, eloquence, and sociability commonly associated with drinking are due not to stimulation but to the initial depression of regions of the brain that ordinarily inhibit or govern such feelings and behavior. Such loosening of controls and judgment accounts for alcohol's legendary use as an *aphrodisiac*, or sexual stimulant: social inhibitions and concerns about sexual behavior are relaxed after drinking, and drinkers may become bolder and more flirtatious.

Higher levels of alcohol in the blood cause further depression of the central nervous system. Rational thought, memory, speech, vision, balance, and coordination are disrupted. This frequently leads to accidents such as falls or burns and, more tragically, traffic injuries or fatalities caused by drunk drivers. Intoxication with alcohol can cause rapid mood swings, aggression, and violence. At very high levels, acute alcohol poisoning occurs: the drinker loses consciousness, has severe breathing problems, and may die in the absence of immediate medical intervention. Dangerous respiratory depression and coma occur more easily when alcohol is mixed with other depressants, such as barbiturates and minor tranquilizers such as Valium.

Chronic Effects

Long-term heavy drinking leads to a variety of further serious problems. Malnutrition such as vitamin deficiencies can occur from poor eating habits and from the effects of ethanol on the stomach and food absorption. This in turn can cause severe brain disturbances and permanent damage known as *encephalopathies* and *psychoses*. Memory and sleep can be disrupted. The liver, one of the body's most important organs, can become enlarged with fat; *cirrhosis*, a chronic and ultimately fatal disease of the liver, can occur. Alcohol affects heart muscle and is a major cause of *cardiomyopathy*, a serious form of heart disease. Chronic heavy drinking leads to tolerance and extreme withdrawal symptoms such as tremors, nausea, sleep disturbances, hallucinations, and possibly death.

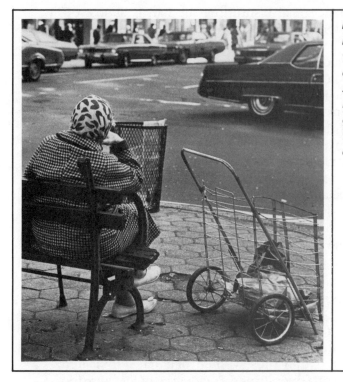

Loneliness is a major reason that some women turn to alcohol, but this solution may only mask, and possibly complicate, underlying feelings of depression and inadequacy.

Women With Drinking Problems

Although there are conflicting reports on the actual degree of increase in female drinking in recent years, few researchers doubt that it has risen over the last few decades. Not unexpectedly, most studies reveal important differences between men and women in almost all aspects of alcohol abuse — its causes, patterns, and consequences.

In general, women with alcohol problems start drinking later than men; actual problem drinking starts during the early or mid-30s although it may begin earlier in unmarried women. This gender difference may be fading away, however, as more and more women — like their male counterparts — commence drinking in their teens.

Another important difference is that most male alcoholics do much of their drinking socially, whereas most female alcoholics tend to drink alone in the privacy (or secrecy) of their homes; as noted earlier, drinking by women is simply not considered as socially acceptable as men's drinking. One important social institution, the bar, is almost off limits to many women, who dare not enter alone for fear of being considered promiscuous and/or alcoholic. Married women, unmarried employed women, and women of high socioeconomic status are especially likely to drink by themselves. Such behavior is probably closely linked to the desire to hide one's drinking, often out of fear of jeopardizing one's marriage, job, or financial security.

Moreover, many women drink to escape emotional problems such as anxiety, depression, and unhappiness. They, more than men, seem to turn to alcohol after traumatic life events and especially after psychological losses such as divorce, death of a spouse or other family members, loss of job, or illness. Other problems, such as unplanned pregnancies, abortions, and the onset of menopause, also may lead to increased drinking.

Special Effects in Women

Because women tend to weigh less and contain relatively more body fat than men, alcohol remains in the bloodstream for a longer period, and thus women become intoxicated more quickly and on fewer drinks. The degree of intoxication seems also to vary with hormonal changes during the menstrual cycle, so that alcohol's effects in women are strongest just before menstruation and weakest just after menstruation. Heavy drinking may also disrupt the menstrual cycle and cause such problems as decreased interest in sex and loss of sexual pleasure. Alcohol consumption by pregnant women can also damage the fetus, an issue discussed in Chapter 8.

Polydrug Abuse

Studies indicate that women are more likely than men to mix other drugs with alcohol, partially because a greater number of women use prescription drugs such as sedatives, tranquilizers, and amphetamines. Marijuana, cocaine, and other illicit drugs may also be abused in combination with alcohol. Mixing other central nervous system depressants such as barbiturates, sleeping pills, or Valium with alcohol is extremely dangerous and is in fact a common method employed by women attempting suicide.

Consequences of Female Alcoholism

In addition to the health problems discussed above, women alcoholics can face a variety of other issues. Here too there are significant gender differences: male alcoholics tend to have problems at work, while women who abuse alcohol seem to have more troubles with family life. Relationships with one's spouse can of course suffer dramatically as a result of problem drinking. Sexual relations can suffer, and this, the actual drinking, and possible extramarital affairs by either spouse may cause serious marital discord, domestic violence, and separation or divorce. In addition, many women alcoholics are married to heavy drinkers, which serves only to aggravate the situation.

Children can suffer from their mothers' drinking in many ways. Alcoholic mothers are often incapable of taking proper care of their children: child neglect is not unusual, and the

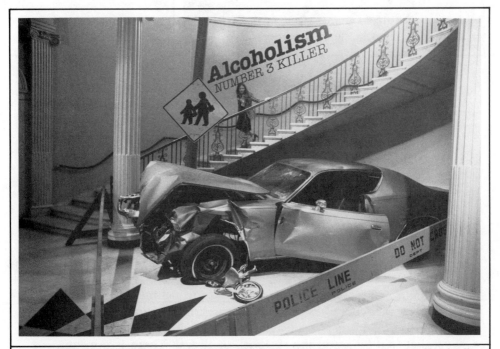

A museum display illustrates the hazards of alcohol abuse. Half of all automobile accidents are alcohol-related. This danger is particularly associated with heavy drinking among young people.

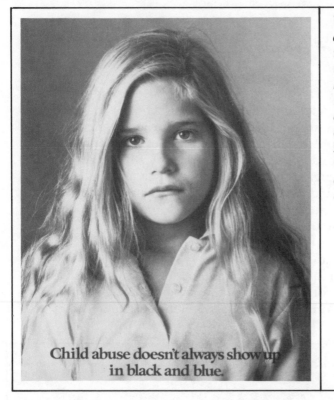

Child abuse doesn't always show up
in black and blue.

The families of alcoholics are among the primary victims of this disease. Alcoholic mothers often neglect their children and may even abuse them. The children are themselves sometimes led at a very early age to abuse alcohol and other drugs.

whole syndrome of frustration, rage, and feelings of helplessness that accompany alcoholism may lead to child abuse. Serious emotional and behavioral problems can develop in children with one or more alcoholic parent, and there is much evidence to suggest that these children are much more likely to go on to abuse alcohol and other drugs themselves. Curiously, it seems that daughters are more influenced in this way than sons, especially by an alcoholic mother.

Teenage Women and Alcohol

Alcohol poses special problems for teenagers, and especially for young women. For one thing, it is readily available from friends, older siblings, parents' liquor cabinets, or liquor stores. Many families permit some degree of drinking by their children, and response to a teenage alcohol problem is often relief that "it's nothing serious" or illegal. There is constant peer pressure to use alcohol at parties or within other social groups, even where other drug use is not encouraged or accepted.

The teenage years are times of great social activity, much of it involving cars, sexual experimentation, and alcohol, often in combination. Although boys are more likely to drive while intoxicated than girls, the latter are often passengers and may not criticize drunk driving for fear of alienating themselves from a certain social group or a particular romantic interest.

Teenage alcohol use can cause a variety of other serious problems involving school, family, friends, and other drugs, but perhaps its greatest hazard for young women involves sexual activity. Alcohol is frequently used for purposes of seduction, and many women find themselves sexually involved with or even violated by men while intoxicated. This can have various negative results — including sexually transmitted disease, depression, loss of self-esteem, and further drinking — but needless to say an unwanted pregnancy is the worst hangover a young woman can wake up with.

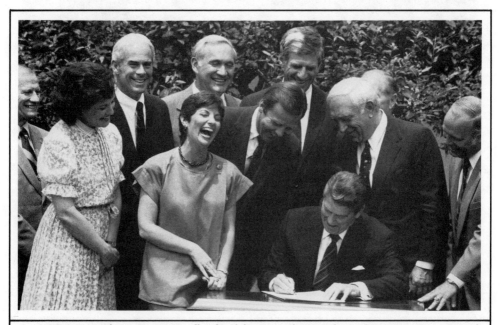

In 1984 President Reagan, flanked by members of Mothers Against Drunk Driving, signed a resolution urging states to make the minimum drinking age 21. The low price and wide acceptance of alcohol make it attractive to young people, who are often ignorant of its dangers.

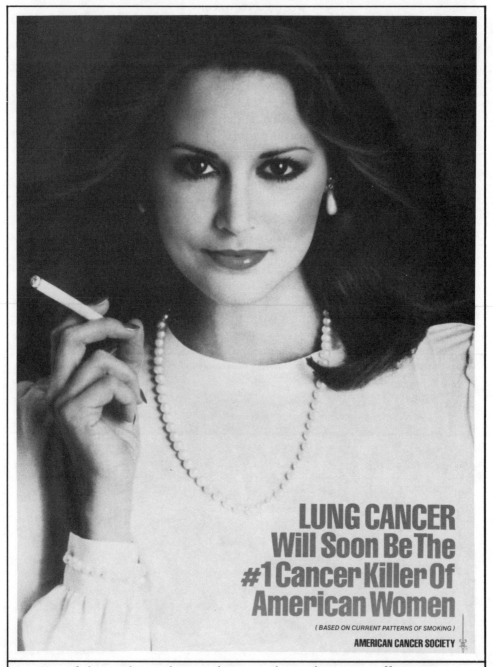

LUNG CANCER Will Soon Be The #1 Cancer Killer Of American Women

(BASED ON CURRENT PATTERNS OF SMOKING)

AMERICAN CANCER SOCIETY

In spite of the evidence that smoking can have disastrous effects on health, the number of women smokers is increasing. Women suffer as much as men from the health hazards of smoking, and women who smoke during pregnancy run the additional risk of damaging their babies.

CHAPTER 3

WOMEN AND CIGARETTES

Like alcohol, tobacco is a psychoactive substance that is just as hazardous as many illicit drugs but whose use is nonetheless legal and generally socially accepted. Although the powerful tobacco industry continuously attempts to convince the public otherwise, it has been firmly and scientifically established that smoking harms one's health in a number of ways. Cigarette smoking has been described as the largest preventable cause of death in the United States.

General Features of Cigarettes

There are more than 4,000 chemical compounds present in cigarette smoke. The exact content depends upon such factors as the brand and length of the cigarette and the type of filter (if any). Rapid smoking produces higher temperatures at the lit end of the cigarette, which can form new compounds. The so-called "sidestream smoke," or that which goes immediately into the environment, is completely unfiltered and can be especially hazardous to the bystander or "passive smoker."

Nicotine, Tar, and Carbon Monoxide

The most dangerous components of cigarette smoke are nicotine, tar, and carbon monoxide. Nicotine has widespread effects throughout the body and accounts for the mood changes caused by smoking as well as the habit's extreme

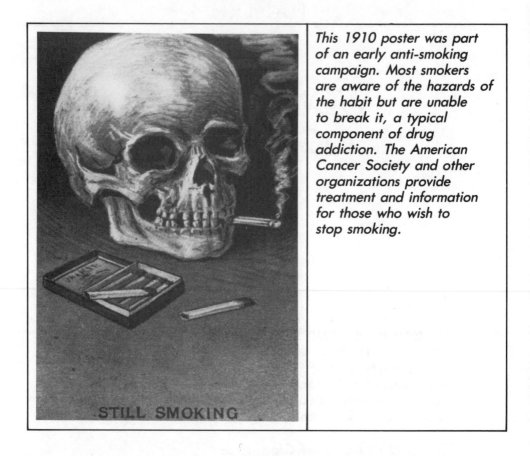

STILL SMOKING

This 1910 poster was part of an early anti-smoking campaign. Most smokers are aware of the hazards of the habit but are unable to break it, a typical component of drug addiction. The American Cancer Society and other organizations provide treatment and information for those who wish to stop smoking.

addictiveness. Nicotine's general effects are due primarily to its actions at the *ganglia*, which are junctions found all over the nervous system.

The nicotine in tobacco smoke acts on the nervous system to produce a variety of complex results, both directly and by causing the release of the powerful chemical *adrenaline* into the bloodstream. (Adrenaline is normally released at times of stress — so-called fight or flight situations — to increase heart rate and blood flow to muscles, among other effects.) Thus nicotine usually causes a faster pulse and raised blood pressure. Actions on the gastrointestinal (digestive) system can cause nausea, vomiting, and diarrhea, particularly in first-time smokers unused to nicotine's effects. Vomiting may also be caused by nicotine's direct stimulation of an area in the brain known as the *chemoreceptor trigger zone* that controls the vomiting reflex.

The effects of nicotine within the central nervous system are complicated and not yet completely understood. Nicotine can cause tremors and, at high doses, convulsions. Actions on the respiration center may lead to stimulation followed by depression of breathing. Acute nicotine poisoning can occur, usually in children, causing a variety of symptoms ranging from nausea, vomiting, and diarrhea to mental disturbances, convulsions, respiratory failure, and death.

The nicotine component of cigarette smoke is probably responsible for other effects of smoking on the brain. Studies have shown that it has specific effects on mood and mental activity, including a decrease in appetite and irritability, muscle relaxant effects, facilitation of memory and attention, and an increase in alertness.

Tar is a general name for the particles left in cigarette smoke after nicotine and moisture have been removed. As its fairly unattractive name suggests, "tar" contains several hazardous substances. Chemicals termed *polycyclic aromatic hydrocarbons* are perhaps most important; one of these, benzopyrene, is a powerful *carcinogen*, or cancer-causing substance. Tar can also contain radioactive particles such as polonium 210.

Carbon monoxide, a small molecule consisting of only two atoms, carbon and oxygen, is another poison contained in cigarette smoke. Every cell in the body continuously requires oxygen, which is transported in the bloodstream by red blood cells. These are specialized to carry oxygen from the lungs throughout the body; this is achieved by the binding of oxygen molecules (O_2) to the vital hemoglobin molecules inside red blood cells. Carbon monoxide (CO), however, binds much more easily and powerfully to hemoglobin than does oxygen; inhalation of carbon monoxide thus lessens the amount of oxygen carried in the bloodstream. This can lead to various degrees of *hypoxia*, or lack of oxygen, a condition that can damage tissues and, at high doses, cause death.

Long-term Effects

Most people know that smoking is a prime cause of cancer. The carcinogenic qualities of cigarette smoke are well established and are due mainly to the tar content. Lung cancers are best known, but smoking has been linked to cancers of the mouth, larynx, esophagus, bladder, and pancreas. What

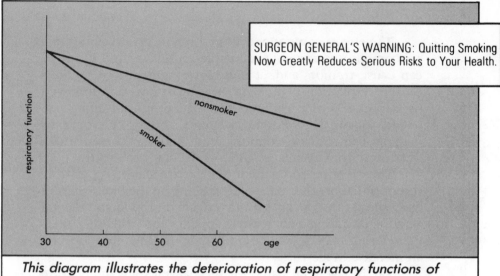

SURGEON GENERAL'S WARNING: Quitting Smoking Now Greatly Reduces Serious Risks to Your Health.

This diagram illustrates the deterioration of respiratory functions of smokers as compared to nonsmokers. The effects of smoking increase considerably with age and the number of years the habit has lasted.

many people are not aware of, however, is that cigarette smoking can also lead to a number of other serious health problems.

Chronic smoking dangerously interferes with the supply of blood to the heart and brain (the cardiovascular and cerebrovascular systems). This can result in *coronary artery disease*, which can cause heart attacks and disabling or fatal cerebrovascular accidents, also known as strokes. Nicotine and carbon monoxide can upset the heart's natural rhythm. Smoking increases the tendency of blood to clot, which causes *atherosclerosis*, or "hardening of the arteries."

As can be imagined, smoking causes severe damage to the lungs and respiratory system. It has been firmly linked with chronic *bronchitis* and *emphysema*, two serious and potentially crippling lung diseases. Destruction of lung tissue by tobacco smoke can lead to such breathlessness on exertion that the victim can walk only a few steps before pausing for breath.

Special Effects on Women

Similar to statistics concerning alcohol, there is evidence that an increasing number of women are smoking. By and large, women suffer from the same hazards of smoking as do men.

Moreover, in addition to the effects of nicotine on the developing fetus, which are discussed in Chapter 8, tobacco use poses special health problems for women.

Recent evidence suggests that smoking may damage the ovaries and affect hormone release vital to the control of menstruation and pregnancy. There seems to be an earlier age of onset of menopause in women smokers, possibly as a result of such damage.

Women using oral contraceptives (birth control pills) face a special danger from smoking. It appears that smoking combines with the effects of oral contraceptives to reduce blood levels of an important natural substance called *prostacyclin*, which acts to maintain blood fluidity and prevent unnecessary clotting. Because of this blood "thickening," women who both smoke and use oral contraceptives have an increased risk of heart attacks and strokes. So great is the

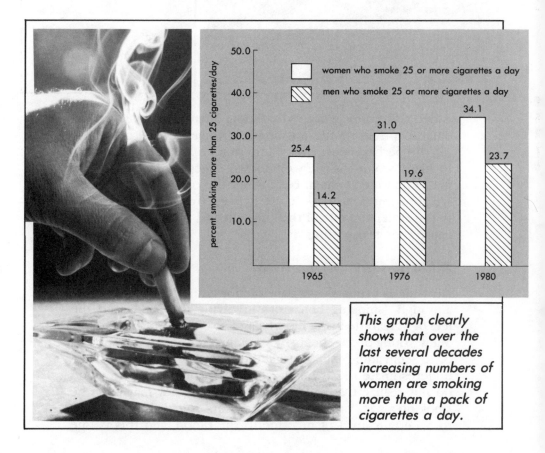

This graph clearly shows that over the last several decades increasing numbers of women are smoking more than a pack of cigarettes a day.

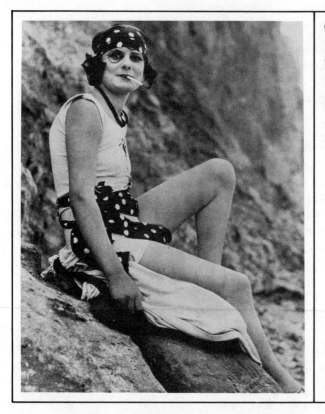

Cigarette and monocle were vital accessories for a thoroughly modern British girl of the 1920s. Tobacco companies have for decades marketed cigarettes as fashionable status symbols.

added risk from cigarettes that some doctors believe that oral contraceptives should not be prescribed for smokers.

Of perhaps less medical importance but of great concern to many women is the well-known effect of smoking on appetite and metabolism. Because of the obsession with their weight, some continue — or perhaps even commence — smoking in order to control their weight and put off quitting because they fear getting "fat."

Addiction and Withdrawal

Nicotine is primarily responsible for addiction to cigarettes, although "smoking behavior" involving the hands and the feel of a cigarette in the mouth can also become habit forming. Many young people begin by smoking a few cigarettes socially or to seem adult, thinking that they can quit at any time. They underestimate the strongly addictive nature of nicotine and do not realize that as tolerance develops they may soon be smoking a pack or more a day. Smokers quickly become used to a certain level of nicotine in the blood, and this is one problem with "low tar and nicotine" cigarettes: the lower amounts of nicotine in each cigarette cause the smoker to inhale more deeply and more often and even to smoke more cigarettes to feed his or her nicotine habit.

Withdrawal from nicotine addiction is difficult and is complicated by a variety of unpleasant withdrawal symptoms. Unfortunately, these may be severe enough to persuade a would-be quitter to return to smoking. Such symptoms can include craving, anxiety, irritability, and difficulty in concentrating. Drowsiness, headaches, increased appetite, gastrointestinal disturbances, and sleeping difficulties also occur. In general, women seem to report more withdrawal difficulties than men, but this may be because men tend not to be as vocal as women about physical problems.

Although no easy method of quitting has yet been developed, studies suggest that stopping abruptly reduces the degree and duration of withdrawal symptoms. This may account for the greater reported success rate of those who stop "cold turkey" than of those who try to "taper off" their smoking. Of course, it is easiest simply never to start.

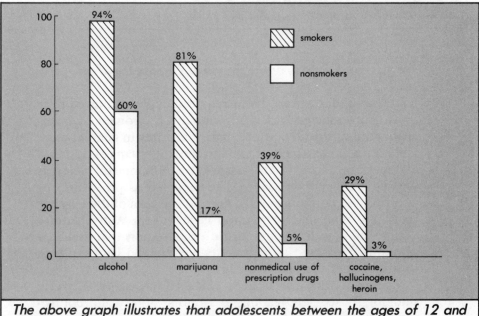

The above graph illustrates that adolescents between the ages of 12 and 17 who smoke are more inclined than their nonsmoking peers to use psychoactive substances such as marijuana, alcohol, and cocaine.

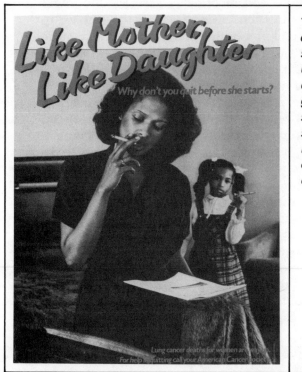

Like Mother, Like Daughter

Why don't you quit before she starts?

Lung cancer deaths for women are rising.
For help in quitting call your American Cancer Society.

"Like mother, like daughter." Parents who smoke endanger their unborn offspring and can do damage to their growing children. Studies show that the children of smokers are more likely to indulge in this highly addictive habit than are the children of nonsmokers.

Trends and Patterns in Female Cigarette Use

Just as attitudes toward women's drinking have altered over this century, society's views on smoking by women have also changed dramatically. At one time cigarettes in general were looked upon negatively: men who smoked them (as opposed to cigars or pipes) were regarded as effeminate, whereas women smokers were viewed suspiciously as prostitutes or of otherwise dubious morals. Around the turn of the century an Illinois woman, Lucy Gaston Page, led the Anti-Cigarette League of America, a moralistic organization that attacked smoking, stressing that it was degenerate and likely to lead to other vices such as drinking.

After World War I there was an increase in cigarette smoking by women, leading to a public outcry and controversy. Women could be arrested for smoking in public during the early 1920s; however, that had changed by the end of the decade. As a *New York Times* headline proclaimed on

August 8, 1927: "Woman No Longer Hides Her Cigarette: She Now Finds She Can Smoke Anywhere."

This theme of women's "liberation" and "freedom" to smoke has been cleverly exploited in our own time by the tobacco industry, as typified by the famous Virginia Slims advertising campaign: "You've Come a Long Way, Baby." As with most cigarette advertisements aimed at women, these almost invariably picture a young, attractive, and obviously successful woman holding a very "feminine" cigarette. Interestingly, these models look as though they have never smoked a cigarette in their lives: their vibrant and healthy looks stand in ironic contrast to the dull complexion, the coughing, tobacco breath, nicotine-stained teeth and fingers, ash burns, and disease caused by cigarette smoking.

Advertisements portraying the female smoker as slender, attractive, and sophisticated seem to have worked. Whereas smoking by men has steadily declined over the last few decades, it has risen among women; women actually surpass men in the "pack-a-day" group. Studies show that among teenagers more girls smoke than boys. In addition, whereas male smokers today tend to be less educated and of lower than average socioeconomic status, women smokers are generally better educated and earn good salaries. This may be yet another effect of women's recent entry into the workplace and the adoption of habits once reserved for men.

Given the evidence that children of smokers are much more likely to smoke than those of nonsmokers, increased smoking by adult women is probably causing more daughters to smoke cigarettes. This point has important repercussions with regard to other drug use, as teenagers who smoke cigarettes are also more likely to experiment with marijuana and other substances.

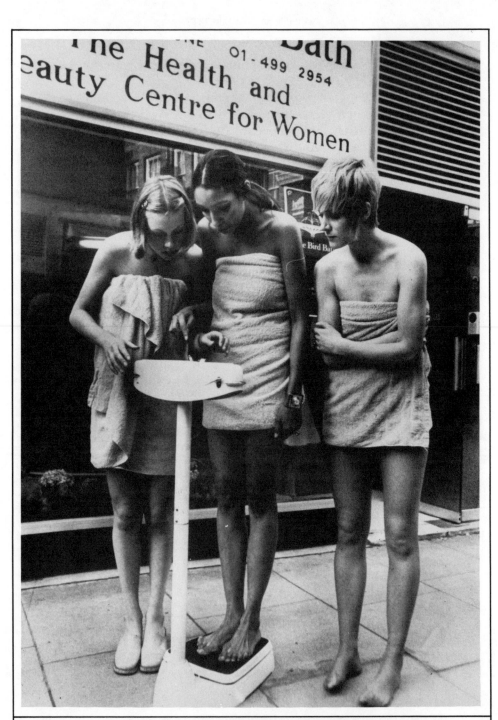

Three women check the scale after exercising. Stimulants curb the appetite and are attractive to many women preoccupied with dieting.

CHAPTER 4

WOMEN AND STIMULANTS

Substances that increase central nervous system activity and alertness, decrease fatigue, and produce euphoria (a strong feeling of elation) are known as stimulants. Because these drugs influence the activity of the important neurotransmitters throughout the body, they also cause other — and sometimes fatal — changes in heart rate, blood pressure, and other systems. Many drugs, even common ones such as caffeine, fall into the stimulant category, but only the two most commonly abused — amphetamines and cocaine — are considered here. As with most drugs, there are special concerns and hazards associated with use by women of these substances, not least because a recent survey of high-school students found that stimulants were the only illicit substances used by more female than male students.

Amphetamines

The family of drugs known as amphetamines is sold under many names and called by a variety of nicknames — most commonly "speed." Commercial names such as Benzedrine, Methedrine, and Dexedrine and street names like bennies, dexies, pep pills, and uppers all refer to amphetamines or their derivatives, and all cause similar effects on the user.

Because stimulants generally work by causing or prolonging the release of specific neurotransmitters from nerve endings, they affect chemical actions not only in the brain but throughout the body. Amphetamines are extremely powerful *sympathomimetics*: these are substances stimulating the sympathetic nervous system, which governs heart rate, blood pressure, and blood flow throughout the body. Thus amphetamines increase blood pressure, change heart rate, and, in large doses, can cause serious cardiac *arrhythmias* (disruption of normal heart rhythm). Gastrointestinal effects can include nausea, vomiting, and diarrhea. Additionally, because amphetamines cause the muscles controlling the opening of the bladder to contract, users may feel pain and have difficulty urinating.

The main effect of amphetamines on the central nervous system is powerful stimulation: amphetamines elevate mood, increase alertness, reduce fatigue, enhance self-confidence, and increase motor and speech activity. Athletic performance may be improved, which leads to abuse among athletes. Amphetamine users often believe that their mental performance is enhanced as well; however, while simple tasks may be performed more rapidly, accuracy is rarely increased.

Amphetamines are well-known *anorectics*, drugs that suppress appetite. Eating behavior is partly controlled by two areas in a part of the brain known as the *hypothalamus*: the feeding center governs appetite and feelings of hunger; the satiety center is responsible for the feeling of being "full" and satisfied after a meal. Amphetamines seem to influence the feeding center and thus reduce the appetite. Tolerance rapidly develops to this anorectic effect, however, and weight loss from amphetamines is short-term (two to four weeks). Most doctors discourage such dietary use.

The harmful effects of most stimulants are both physiological and psychological. These problems can occur at almost any dose, depending on the user. Intravenous use, which leads to powerful "rushes" and more frequent use at higher doses, is especially dangerous. (Intravenous users also face the deadly risks of all drug use involving needles: hepatitis, AIDS, and other transmitted diseases. See Chapter 7.) Amphetamines can cause nausea, vomiting, and diarrhea.

Symptoms of acute amphetamine poisoning, which occurs after an overdose and can be fatal, include dizziness, tremors, paranoid hallucinations, panic, suicidal and homicidal tendencies, and extreme fatigue and depression. Use of

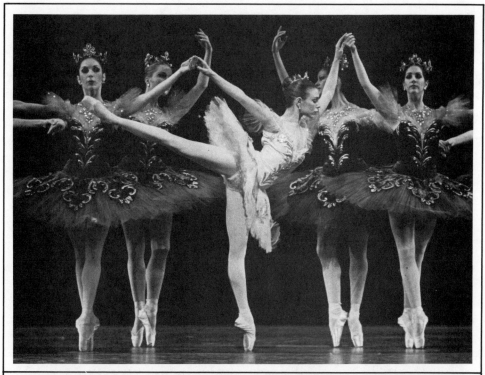

Gelsey Kirkland, a principal dancer of the American Ballet Theatre, recently confessed to a long period of cocaine addiction.

these stimulants can also lead to cardiac arrhythmias and extreme shifts in blood pressure, conditions that can result in death. The acute effects listed above can occur in any user after a long period of use. Long-term amphetamine abuse leads to increased mental disturbance and weight loss. Psychosis, vivid hallucinations, and paranoia are most common. Mechanical, repetitive behavior, such as repeatedly taking apart small objects, can also occur.

As with many other drugs, a great problem of amphetamine abuse is that tolerance to its effects occurs rapidly. To continue achieving a euphoric "high," or to continue appetite suppression, users must continually increase the dose. Many people begin with small doses — for social and recreational use, to reduce fatigue while studying or to improve athletic performance, or for weight loss — and eventually become dependent on it. However, tolerance does not develop to some of amphetamines' effects on the brain, and increased doses and use can lead to serious mental disturbance.

Women and Amphetamines

That stimulants such as amphetamines are the only illicit drugs used by more high school girls than boys is certainly due in part to the traditional use of amphetamines as appetite suppressants. Although, as noted earlier, research has shown that the anorectic effect of this drug tends to last only four weeks at most, many young women still turn to these pills thinking that they offer a quick and painless solution to their weight problems. After tolerance develops to the appetite suppressant effects, increased doses may be taken in an attempt to continue with weight loss. Soon a full-blown addiction can occur, and the victims of this dependency will find that weight loss is the least of their concerns.

Because amphetamines combat fatigue and increase physical activity, some housewives use them to help survive a hectic day. Many women who abuse alcohol, barbiturates, Valium, or other central nervous system depressants take

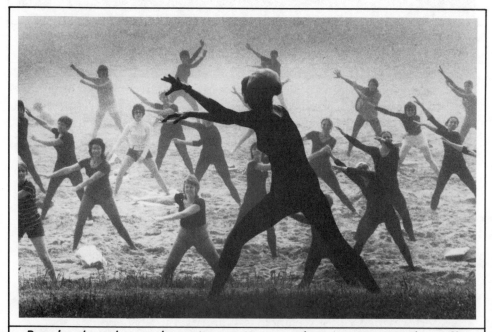

People who take amphetamines to increase their energy can also suffer side effects such as nausea and diarrhea. Regular exercise provides the good effects of stimulants without the unpleasant consequences.

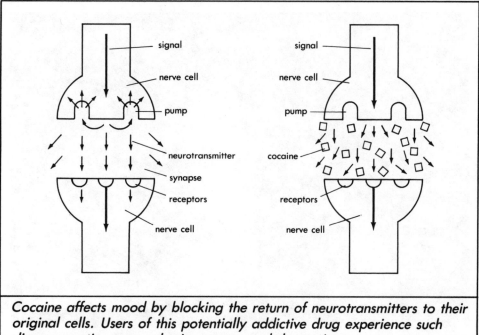

signal

nerve cell

pump

neurotransmitter

synapse

receptors

nerve cell

signal

nerve cell

pump

cocaine

receptors

nerve cell

Cocaine affects mood by blocking the return of neurotransmitters to their original cells. Users of this potentially addictive drug experience such diverse emotions as euphoria, anger, and depression.

"uppers" to wake them up after their "downer" of the night before. Such dependence on drugs to regulate normal sleeping and waking cycles is the sign of a serious "polydrug" abuse problem.

Cocaine

Cocaine has been called "the drug of the eighties" and the "ultimate high." It has also been labeled harmless and non-addictive. As greater supply, reduced prices, and a glamorous image have led to increased use of "coke" among all ages (while use of marijuana and some other drugs has declined), it has become very clear that cocaine is far from harmless and is quite possibly the most addictive drug in current use. A new form of cocaine known as "crack" is more powerful and easier to obtain, creating more addicts than ever before.

The effects of cocaine are essentially similar to those of amphetamines, which is not surprising, since it acts to increase the activity of the same vital neurotransmitters, although in a different way. Under normal circumstances, when

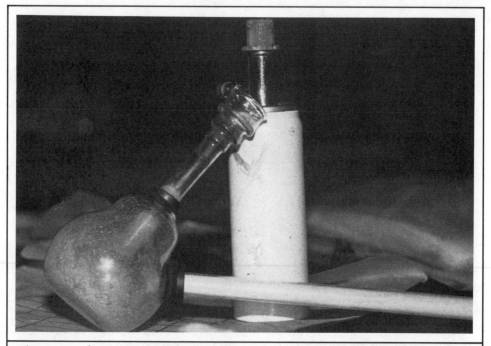

This type of pipe is used for smoking crack, a crude, extremely addictive form of cocaine. The abuse of all forms of cocaine has penetrated every economic and social level of society.

these neurotransmitters (three important ones are dopamine, serotonin, and norepinephrine) are released from a nerve ending to bind to their receptors on another nerve cell, their action is limited by the reuptake (or reabsorption) of the chemicals back into the nerve ending. Cocaine works by blocking this reuptake, and thus the released neurotransmitters act for longer periods. Effects of cocaine are similar to those of amphetamines and include feelings of euphoria, increased alertness, and an increase in heart rate and blood pressure. Heavy use of the drug, however, leads to the depletion of neurotransmitter reserves, which can cause extreme depression, the very opposite of cocaine's pleasurable effect.

Indeed, cocaine has definite negative and even fatal effects. The short-lived euphoria can lead to a severe depression or "crash." The most serious result of acute cocaine poisoning involves the drug's effects on the heart and blood vessels.

Because cocaine can greatly and rapidly increase heart rate and blood pressure, it can cause fatal heart attacks and strokes. Chronic use can lead to insomnia, weight loss, irritability, paranoia, and psychosis. All of cocaine's harmful physiological and psychological side effects, as well as addiction, can occur not only from injecting or smoking it, but also from inhaling it. Other possibly fatal side effects can result from the various substances used to "cut" or dilute cocaine for sale in order to maximize profits. None of the cocaine sold on the street is remotely pure.

Crack and Freebasing

Ordinary pure cocaine powder is really a salt form of the drug known scientifically as cocaine hydrochloride. The freebasing technique is a simple chemical reaction that produces a modified form, cocaine base. This is now sold cheaply (often for only $5 or $10) as small pellets called crack which when smoked gives an immediate and short-lasting high. (The smoked cocaine base gets to the brain more quickly than the inhaled cocaine salt.) It should be noted that crack is an extremely addictive and potentially dangerous drug.

Addiction to Cocaine

As noted, cocaine was for many years considered nonaddictive and "safe." This view, which was based on a traditional scientific definition of addiction involving the concepts of tolerance and withdrawal symptoms, is now entirely discredited. Indeed, cocaine causes extreme psychological addiction. This dependency is linked to the apparent direct effects of the drug on the brain's "pleasure center" and possibly involves the neurotransmitter dopamine. Several experiments have demonstrated cocaine's addictiveness, which seems even more powerful than that of heroin: in one test, monkeys who were given the choice between food and cocaine for eight days invariably chose the drug. In another experiment, trained rats would push a lever 2,000 times to get heroin—and up to 12,000 times to get cocaine.

Other features of cocaine cause problems of addiction. Unlike one's first experience of many drugs (for example, tobacco, alcohol, or marijuana), where the effects may be negative or simply unnoticeable, the first use of cocaine is

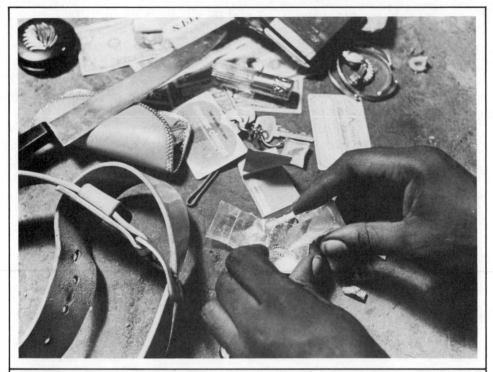

Cocaine and equipment for its use are found among the spilled contents of a woman's purse. The dangerous pharmacological effects of cocaine are essentially the same in women as in men.

almost always pleasurable. Many users still delude themselves that the drug is nonaddictive. The recent crack phenomenon has enabled more young people than ever before to try this powerful drug—and to become addicted.

Women and Cocaine

Unlike some of the drugs discussed so far, the pharmacological effects of cocaine are essentially the same in women as in men (although there may be an effect on the fetus; see Chapter 8). The main difference is social. The tremendously addicting qualities of cocaine lead to a frantic obsession with getting more — and at whatever price. The new crack form of cocaine is markedly cheaper (and more available in some areas) than traditional cocaine powder, but because of its short-lived effects, users need crack even more frequently.

Addicts must have some every thirty minutes or so to avoid the "crash," or severe depression of cocaine withdrawal.

In order to obtain the money needed to sustain their habit, male addicts turn frequently to crime, from petty street theft to high-stakes Wall Street insider trading. Women, however, must often turn to a different, more traditionally female source of money: prostitution. Such is cocaine's addictiveness that many young women find themselves performing sexual acts — sometimes in "coke dens" or nightclub bathrooms — simply to be paid in cocaine, not even in cash. These cocaine users thus face not only the dangers of the drug, but also such hazards of prostitution as physical abuse, pregnancy, venereal disease, and AIDS.

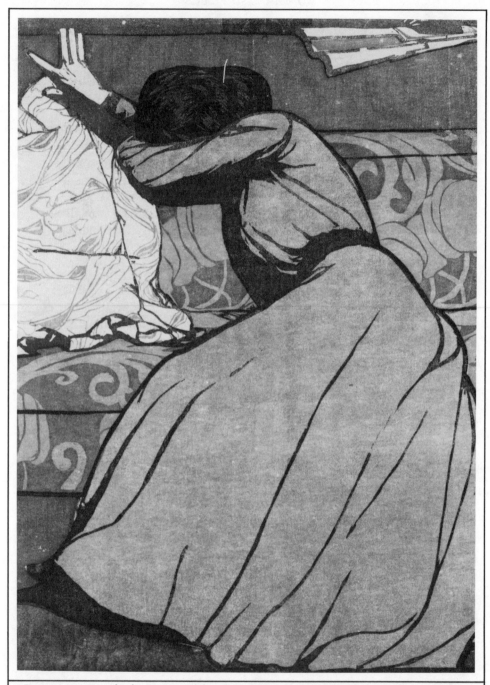

Depressants, which are used by far more women than men, are typically prescribed to alleviate sleeplessness and anxiety. Unfortunately, these drugs are both psychologically and physically addictive.

CHAPTER 5

WOMEN AND DEPRESSANTS

Drugs such as barbiturates, Quaaludes, and Valium have effects opposite to those of stimulants such as cocaine and amphetamines in that they depress the central nervous system. This action causes drowsiness and facilitates sleep, relaxes one's mood, diminishes concentration, and reduces muscle tone and coordination. Control of heart rate and breathing is also affected, sometimes fatally. Depressants termed "minor" tranquilizers or *anxiolytics*, of which Valium is the best known, are commonly prescribed by doctors to reduce anxiety, sleeplessness, and stress.

Despite the often sensationalist media coverage of the use of "hard" drugs such as cocaine and heroin, depressant abuse is more common. About one in five young people has used this type of drug nonmedically. Abuse of these substances and its problems — including extreme addiction, overdose, and withdrawal symptoms — is of special concern to women, who, according to statistics, use these drugs far more often than men.

Depressants are members of several drug families and go by a variety of names. Medically they are referred to as minor tranquilizers, sedatives, hypnotics, and antianxiety (or anxiolytic) drugs. Common names include sleeping pills and trade names such as Valium, Librium, Equanil, Nembutal, Seconal, and Quaalude. (Although Quaaludes are no longer manufactured by any legitimate pharmaceutical companies, "bootleg" varieties are sometimes available.) On the street, depressants — especially barbiturates — have many nicknames: downers, blues, red devils, yellow jackets, rainbows, and ludes, to name but a few.

The various depressant drugs work by a variety of mechanisms, but all produce the same effect: depression of the central nervous system. As noted in Chapter 2, alcohol is also a central nervous system depressant, so it is not surprising that many of the effects — and hazards — of depressants are similar to those of drinking. One of the most important dangers of depressants is that the effects are additive; mixing any one depressant drug with another, *especially alcohol*, is extremely dangerous and accounts for most drug-based medical emergencies.

Each drug has its own special effects and pharmacological qualities, but the important common features and dangers of the most frequently used depressant drugs are explored below. Particular attention is focused upon barbiturates and benzodiazepines because of their special dangers and widespread abuse among women.

Sedatives and Hypnotics

Various depressants affect the central nervous system in different ways: sedatives relax and calm the user while hypnotics induce sleep. Different brands of these drugs are often advertised for a specific purpose (for either sedative or hypnotic effects), but in general any agent can cause extreme central nervous system depression (coma) at high doses. Some depressants (mainly barbiturates) are used for anesthesia during operations; the benzodiazepines are not anesthetics but are often used medically to relax patients before stressful procedures. Depressants are also used by doctors as muscle relaxants and as anticonvulsants. By far the most common medical use of the benzodiazepines is to reduce anxiety and sleeplessness.

At normal doses most depressants do not cause significant changes in heart function and blood flow. At higher levels, however, they can cause a sharp decrease in blood pressure and increased heart rate.

The effects of depressants — especially barbiturates — on breathing can be very serious. Control of respiration is complicated and involves a *neurogenic* (nerve based) drive in the brain's "respiration center" as well as special chemical

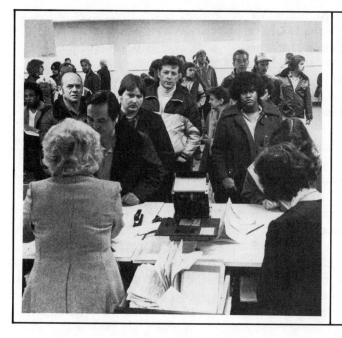

Abuse of tranquilizers and barbiturates is all too common among the unemployed and others who suffer economic hardships.

monitoring of levels of carbon dioxide and oxygen. Barbiturates and other depressants reduce this neurogenic drive, and overdose can lead to respiratory failure and death. Benzodiazepines such as Valium do not significantly affect breathing when taken alone and in normal doses but can do so in combination with alcohol and other depressants.

Many of the mental changes caused by sedatives and tranquilizers are similar to those of alcohol intoxication: confusion, sluggishness, slowness and disorder of thought, slurring of speech, irritability, bad judgment, lack of concentration, and problems with learning and memory. Because these drugs impair motor coordination, driving while under the influence of barbiturates, Valium, or other depressants can be very dangerous. Acute poisoning with depressants occurs most often from barbiturate overdose or from the additive effects of benzodiazepines and alcohol or other depressants, as noted above. The results can include cardiovascular and respiratory depression, coma, pulmonary (lung) complications, renal (kidney) failure, hypothermia (low body temperature), and death.

Barbiturates have long been known to be habit forming, but only recently has the heavily addictive nature of virtually all depressants — including Valium and other benzodiazepines previously considered nonaddictive — been recognized. In search of the depressant "high," addicts use pentobarbital ("yellowjackets"), secobarbital ("red devils"), and many other short-acting (i.e., rapidly effective) barbiturates, as well as methaqualone (Quaaludes) and meprobamate (Miltown, Equanil). The short-acting Valium is preferred by some users to barbiturates.

Addiction can begin either illicitly or after prescribed medical use for stress or insomnia. Alcoholics or users of other drugs will often take barbiturates or benzodiazepines in a misguided attempt to manage the downside of their primary addiction. Heroin users sometimes take depressants to add to the effects of poor-quality street heroin. The combination of barbiturates and amphetamines is reported to cause increased euphoria. The low price and easy availability — depressants can often be found in the household medicine cabinet or a mother's purse — and greater social acceptance of these drugs add to their addictiveness.

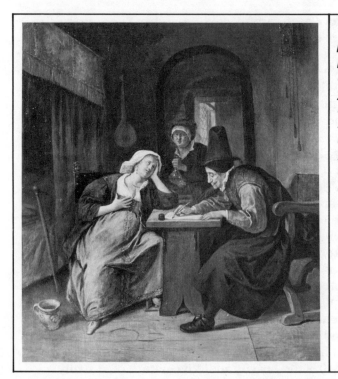

The tendency to treat psychological problems pharmaceutically goes back hundreds of years. Drug companies routinely spend vast sums encouraging doctors to adopt this strategy. Opponents of this method advocate drug-free treatments for stress and anxiety, such as meditation and biofeedback.

The concept of *general depressant withdrawal syndrome* was developed to describe the similar withdrawal symptoms experienced by those addicted to a variety of central nervous system depressants — barbiturates, meprobamate, methaqualone, and benzodiazepines. Mild symptoms include EEG (brain-wave) abnormalities, insomnia and sleep disturbance, and anxiety. More severe withdrawal symptoms may include delirium and seizures, as well as nausea, abdominal cramps, vomiting, headache, paranoid hallucinations, exhaustion, cardiovascular collapse, and even death. With barbiturates, these problems usually begin in the first few days after abstinence and last about eight days. Because of their chemical makeup, benzodiazepines stay in the body longer, and thus withdrawal symptoms may take longer to develop.

Extreme Dangers of the Barbiturates

Barbiturates have a long history of medical use and nonmedical abuse. The development of the benzodiazepines (which cause less respiratory depression when used alone) around 1960 greatly reduced medical use of barbiturates for sedative-hypnotic purposes, but they are still used in anesthesia and anticonvulsant therapy.

Barbiturates are extremely dangerous and account for most deaths from drug overdose each year. One problem is that tolerance to their effects develops quickly, so that doses must be increased in order to achieve the same effects. The lethal dose, however, is not much higher in addicts than in normal users, so even a slightly higher dose than usual may prove fatal. Additionally, *active metabolites* (breakdown products that also have effects) can accumulate in the bloodstream after continual use.

These metabolites are formed by the liver, which handles and detoxifies most drugs, as well as many of the body's own chemical products. Barbiturates increase the speed with which the liver performs these functions by a process known as *hepatic enzyme induction*. Barbiturates also increase the rate at which foreign substances are excreted in the urine. Because of speeded-up liver function, oral contraceptives are broken down more rapidly in women who use barbiturates and are thus less effective. Unwanted pregnancies may therefore occur.

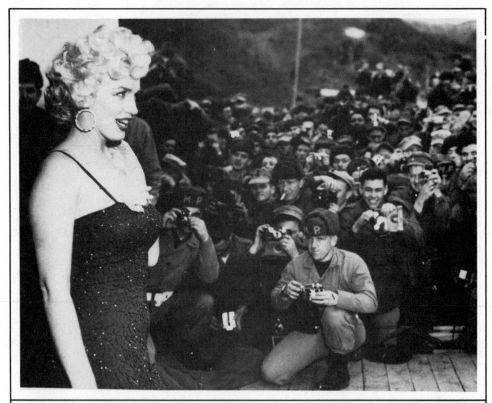

Marilyn Monroe entertains troops during the Korean War. The personification of sexual attraction for an entire generation, Monroe abused barbiturates and died of an overdose while still a young woman.

Benzodiazepines

Statistics provide ample evidence of the immense popularity of the benzodiazepines. Currently there are about 5 million regular cocaine users, 20 million regular marijuana users, and one-half million heroin addicts in the United States. By contrast, in 1980 there were almost 34 million Valium prescriptions written and many more for other benzodiazepines such as Librium, Ativan, and Tranxene. Although heroin, cocaine, and other drugs cause many deaths and medical emergencies, the Drug Abuse Warning Network (DAWN) indicates that Valium overdose is second only to alcohol-and-depressant combinations in causing emergency room entries. In 1981 there were about 3,500 overdoses reported by DAWN for each of the drugs marijuana and cocaine. In 1980 there were more than 16,000 DAWN-reported Valium emergencies.

These facts do not by any means minimize the dangers of other drugs. Instead, they stress the high potential for benzodiazepine abuse. Because minor tranquilizers are so easily available and so widely prescribed, many users — most of whom are women — run the risk of becoming addicted to or overdosing on these central nervous system depressants.

The benzodiazepine drug family currently includes about 25 substances in clinical use around the world as sedative-hypnotics. Modifications of the parent molecule result in changes in strength, speed, and duration of activity. Drug companies like to market different varieties for specific purposes (e.g., one pill to reduce anxiety and another to induce sleep), but this is often only for commercial reasons. Any benzodiazepine can cause significant central nervous system depression after a high dose.

The two most popular benzodiazepines are Valium (or diazepam) and Librium (chlordiazepoxide), both introduced around 1960. Research over the last decade has determined that these drugs work on a benzodiazepine receptor, which

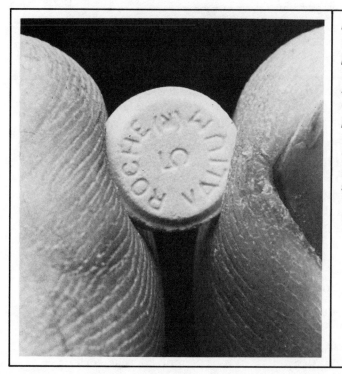

In 1979 Valium was the most widely prescribed drug in the United States. Although sales declined after massive publicity about its long-term effects, the drug is still heavily used. In every age group, twice as many women as men take tranquilizers.

*Drug Abuse Warning Network, which records the causes of emergency visits to 622 cooperating hospitals

when stimulated influences the effects of a general inhibitory neurotransmitter, gamma-aminobutyric acid (GABA), at its own GABA receptors. This action suggests that the body may produce a natural, or *endogenous*, substance that binds to these benzodiazepine receptors to produce the same effects of sedation and sleep.

The "Safe" Tranquilizer?

When first introduced, Valium, Librium and other benzodiazepines were hailed as safe sedative hypnotics. Although it is true that benzodiazepine overdose is usually not as serious as barbiturate overdose, it is now recognized that serious side effects exist. These can include paradoxical effects, such as increased anxiety, irritability, heart rate, and sweating; hallucinations; paranoia; depression; and respiratory depression and coma.

After initial doubt and controversy, the problem of benzodiazepine addiction is now recognized as a serious possible hazard of the routine treatment of anxiety and insomnia with Valium and similar drugs. Here the benzodiazepines are in a special position because of the tremendous influence of the pharmaceutical industry and the enormous profits made from benzodiazepine sales. In addition, patients often accept on faith the notion that any drug prescribed by their doctor cannot be addictive or harmful.

In 1980 the Food and Drug Administration (FDA) ruled that all benzodiazepine prescriptions would have to include a patient package insert (PPI) describing in simple language

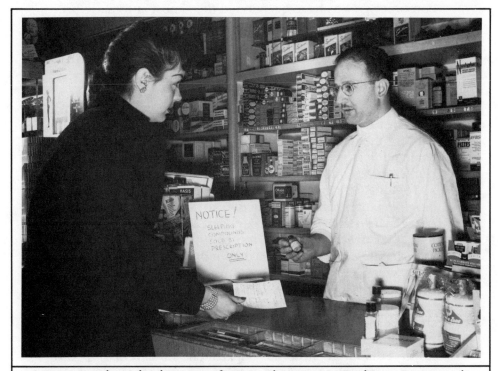

A customer buys barbiturates from a pharmacist. Barbiturates were the most widely prescribed sleeping compounds until the benzodiazepines, depressants with less potential for abuse, appeared in 1960.

the hazards and possible addictiveness of these drugs. After intense lobbying by pharmaceutical companies and the American Medical Association, however, the FDA in 1981 suspended the new rule, which had never been put into force.

Another dangerous side effect of benzodiazepines involves parental (usually maternal) use and the impression it leaves on children. Studies have shown that children whose parents use prescription psychoactive drugs such as Valium are much more likely to experiment with drugs themselves.

Benzodiazepines and Women

This has been a subject of much recent discussion and controversy, and several books and even a film (*I'm Dancing As Fast As I Can*, based on Barbara Gordon's book of the same name) have dealt with the nightmarish problems of women hooked on Valium and similar drugs. Feminist and medical consumer groups have questioned the almost automatic prescription of Valium or one of its "cousins" to any woman complaining of anxiety or sleeplessness. Often women suffering from depression have also been given such drugs. Other prescription drugs (and alcohol) may be used by these patients at the same time, causing further problems.

Although most doctors realize the potential addictive and overdose dangers of benzodiazepines, it is sometimes hard for them to monitor their patients' drug taking properly. Some addicts get prescriptions for Valium or other tranquilizers from several doctors at the same time in order to enlarge and maintain their supply. Initial low "therapeutic" doses that have been prescribed by a doctor can rapidly escalate to daily doses many times stronger. Very real addiction, with the potential for overdose, can all too easily ensue.

Needless to say, doctors do not intend their patients any harm when prescribing these drugs. Many factors combine to impel physicians to prescribe benzodiazepines. These factors include the doctor's training, drug company influence, short consultations, and both the doctor's and the patient's expectations. As one expert, Professor Ian Oswald of the Royal Edinburgh Hospital Department of Psychiatry, said when referring to benzodiazepine treatment of insomnia: "You are trying to please the patient and to tell yourself that you are a kindly, helpful doctor. You know perfectly well that the patient sleeps far more than she says she sleeps, but you want an easy life, you want to feel comfortable inside, and so you write a prescription."

Fortunately, recent appreciation of the dangers of benzodiazepine tranquilizers has led to a decline in prescriptions from a peak in the late 1970s. Medical emergencies caused by these drugs have also decreased in number. Despite these changing statistics, however, the hazards of benzodiazepine abuse persist.

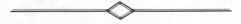

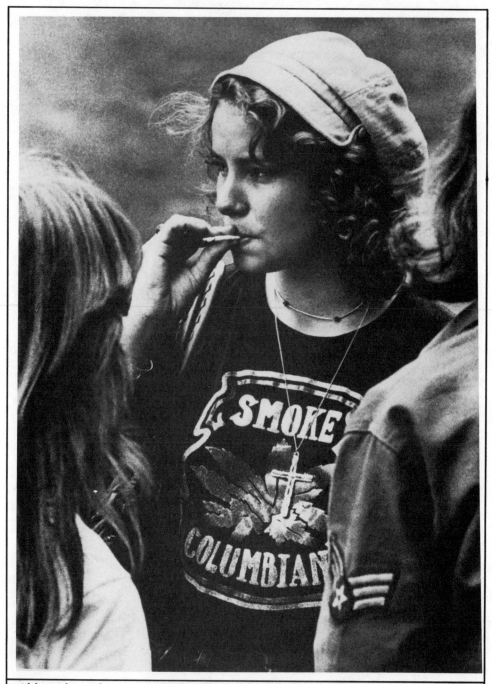

Although evidence concerning the dangers of marijuana has caused its use to decline, a recent study revealed that one-third of the American population over the age of twelve had tried marijuana at least once.

CHAPTER 6

WOMEN AND MARIJUANA

Marijuana and other cannabinoids occupy a unique place among substances of abuse. Although these drugs certainly possess distinct pharmacological qualities, the most important aspect is their widespread use among both men and women, especially among young people. Most high-school and college students are at least exposed to cannabis, often in casual situations such as parties and rock concerts, and more than two-thirds of today's young adults (aged 18 to 25) have tried marijuana at least once.

The potential dangers of cannabinoids are controversial, and some states and nations, acknowledging the popularity and relative safety of cannabis, even allow possession of small amounts of marijuana for personal use. Apart from the possible damaging side effects of cannabis, the persistent — and controversial — question of whether it leads to other drug use is also of concern.

General Features of Marijuana

It is ironic that scientists know less about the actions of the cannabinoids, drugs with such a long history of widespread use, than they do about many other substances. It is known, however, that the active ingredient in derivatives of cannabis is *tetrahydrocannabinol* (THC) and that this chemical is

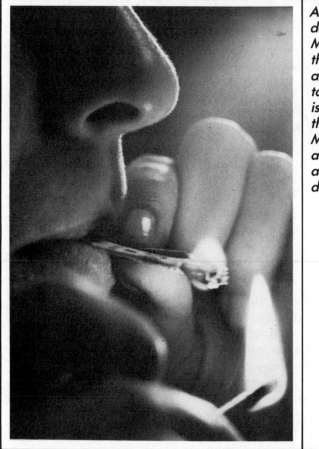

A female smoker inhales deeply on a joint. Marijuana smoking poses the same health hazards as cigarettes; in fact, the tar content of marijuana is more carcinogenic than that of tobacco. Marijuana smoking can also impair coordination and perception, making driving hazardous.

present in varying concentrations in the related substances marijuana, hashish, and other cannabinoids. The following discussion focuses on the actions of marijuana, which is the most popular and widely used cannabinoid. (It is important to note that the potency of marijuana's actions differs according to the concentration of THC in the drug, which can vary from 0.5% to more than 10%.)

The general effects of marijuana include decreased sweating, dry mouth, and other changes related to effects on the neurotransmitter *acetylcholine*. Cannabis also reduces the fluid pressure within the eye (the *intraocular pressure*) and is thus used by some glaucoma sufferers to reduce pain. As marijuana also has *antiemetic* qualities (i.e., it inhibits vomiting), it is sometimes used by patients undergoing radiotherapy or chemotherapy, both of which can cause nausea and vomiting.

Marijuana use can dramatically increase heart rate and blood pressure. When the heart rate is increased, the heart needs additional oxygen. Marijuana increases the amount of carbon monoxide in the blood, which decreases the amount of oxygen delivered to the heart. So although the heart needs more oxygen when a person smokes marijuana, less oxygen than normal is available to it. This situation may be tolerated by a person with a normal heart, but it becomes a serious problem for people with high blood pressure or heart conditions.

Central nervous system effects depend greatly upon the sample's THC content and to a lesser degree on the setting and the user's experience with marijuana. Euphoria, uncontrolled laughter, relaxation, and drowsiness can all occur. Changes in time perception — a general "slowing down" of events — almost always occur. Sensory changes may include enhanced auditory, visual, taste, and tactile sensations. The user's appetite is also frequently stimulated.

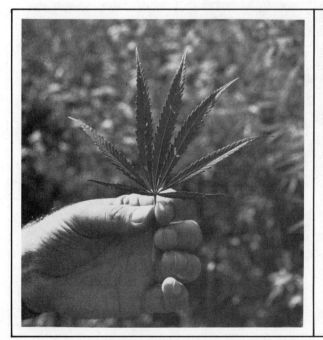

Short-term effects of marijuana include euphoria, drowsiness, and an increase in sensory perceptions. Used over a long period of time, however, the drug can diminish memory, concentration, and learning ability.

Side Effects and Toxicity

Marijuana use can lead to decreased short-term memory, concentration, and learning ability. Driving abilities are also adversely affected, especially when marijuana is used in combination with alcohol. Panic attacks and paranoid reactions are not unusual, especially with regard to the drug's illegality or its use in an unfamiliar setting.

Just as with inhaled tobacco smoke, heavy smoking of marijuana or other cannabis preparations can cause severe lung damage. Although marijuana users generally do not smoke as much as tobacco addicts on a daily basis, marijuana contains many more impurities and can be contaminated with various pesticides. In addition, the tar in marijuana smoke seems to be more carcinogenic than that contained in cigarette smoke.

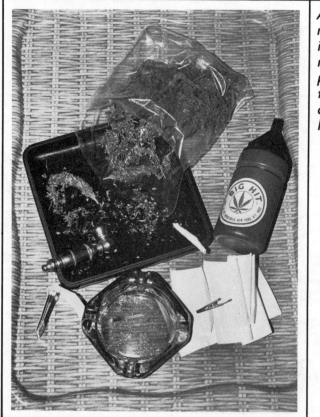

Accessories for marijuana smoking include roach clips, rolling papers, and a pipe. Despite efforts to prohibit them, sales of these items are both legal and profitable.

The psychological and behavioral changes in many long-term and heavy cannabis users are called *amotivational syndrome*. Along with loss of concentration and memory problems, sufferers show compulsive drug-seeking behavior, apathy, and lack of interest in conventional social goals.

As far as addiction and withdrawal are concerned, many researchers consider cannabis only psychologically addicting, because physical tolerance to the drug has not been demonstrated. It seems, however, that abstaining from marijuana after long-term, heavy use can cause such mild withdrawal symptoms as irritability, restlessness, nervousness, weight loss, insomnia, tremor, and chills.

Women, Marijuana, and Other Drug Use

In women who use marijuana regularly, the drug seems to cause menstrual irregularities such as *anovular cycles* (menstrual cycles in which the menstrual flow is not preceded by ovulation).

Although marijuana use among young people in the United States is declining after a peak in the late 1970s, many young men and women still use this common illicit drug. National Institute on Drug Abuse (NIDA) figures for the high-school class of 1984 indicate that marijuana use by women is only slightly less than use by men: 51% of the female students had used it at least once, compared with 58% of the males; use within the previous month was reported by about 21% of the women and 28% of the men.

An interesting recent study of the use of drugs by female college students suggests that marijuana use is associated with further experimentation with other psychoactive substances. There are dramatic differences found in nonmedical drug use between women who use marijuana and those who do not. Use of most other drugs appears to follow rather than precede marijuana use.

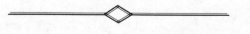

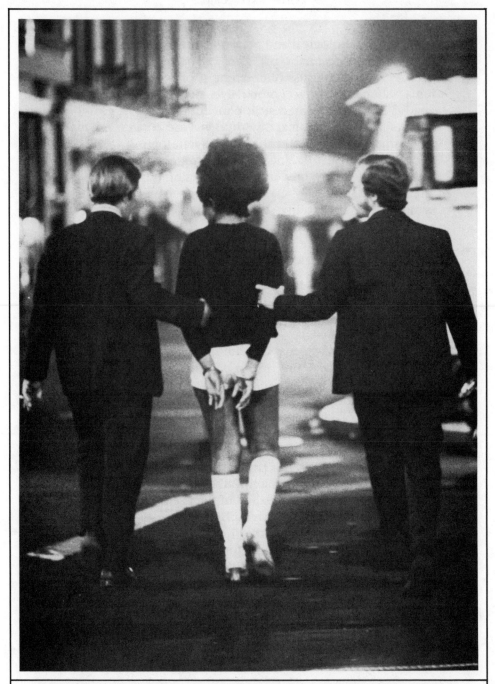

Two plainclothes policemen arrest a young prostitute in New York's notorious Times Square. Some women turn to prostitution and other crimes in a desperate attempt to finance their opiate addictions.

CHAPTER 7

WOMEN AND OPIATES

The group of substances known as opiates (sometimes referred to as narcotics) has a long history of use, both medical and nonmedical. The best-known opiates are heroin and morphine, but other common painkillers such as codeine are also members of the same drug family. Statistically, opiate abuse is relatively uncommon in the United States — there are about 500,000 heroin addicts nationwide — but its dangers are such that heroin addicts rank third in hospital drug emergency admissions.

One of the most important scientific discoveries of recent decades involved the identification of opiate receptors in the human brain. These neurotransmitter receptors are found in a variety of locations in the brain and spinal cord and are stimulated in various ways by substances found in the opium poppy, such as morphine and codeine. Heroin is a synthetic opiate, similar to morphine, which also stimulates opiate receptors. Soon after the discovery of opiate receptors, natural opiates were found in humans. These are the small molecules (known as enkephalins, endorphins, and dynorphins) that act as the natural neurotransmitters at these receptor sites and whose actions are mimicked by heroin and other opiate drugs.

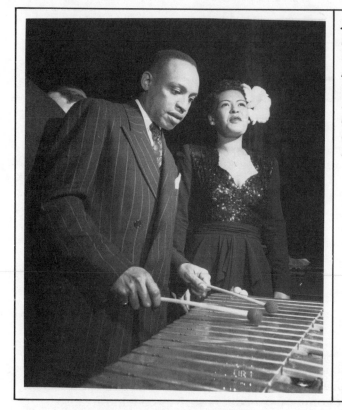

Jazz singer Billie Holiday appeared with Lionel Hampton at the Metropolitan Opera in 1944. Holiday's tragic heroin addiction destroyed her talent and, eventually, her life.

Pain Relief and Euphoria

Opiates have historically been widely used medically as strong analgesics (pain relievers), but other important effects include mood elevation (euphoria), gastrointestinal upset, and, in high doses, coma and death resulting from respiratory depression.

The analgesia caused by opiates is powerful and is the reason for the widespread medical use of morphine in treating pain, especially in patients suffering from cancer and other terminal diseases. Following the discovery of opiate receptors, it was determined that opiates relieve pain because they inhibit the transmission of pain stimuli. This occurs at sites in the spinal cord, where nerve fibers carrying pain impulses meet other fibers going up into the brain.

The other most important effect of opiates on the central nervous system is mood elevation, or euphoria. The basis for the pleasurable "rush" felt by opiate users is not well understood, although it seems to involve a special class of opiate receptors in the brain. Interestingly, not all users (particularly medical patients) achieve this euphoria, especially on first encounter with the drug. Heroin is known to deliver a quicker rush than morphine, because its chemical structure allows it to cross the blood-brain barrier more quickly.

The effects of opiates on the respiratory system account for most deaths from opiate abuse. Heroin, morphine, and other opiates all decrease both the rate and volume of breathing by reducing the brain's response to carbon dioxide levels in the blood. At certain doses, breathing is only accomplished voluntarily — that is, the subject must consciously attempt to draw breath. This respiratory depression increases with the strength of the dose and can lead to coma and death.

Opiates cause constipation by acting on opiate receptors in the bowels to reduce muscular activity and thus slow the passage of food through the gut. Because of this effect, opiates were used medically to treat dysentery (severe diarrhea) many years before their analgesic qualities were exploited.

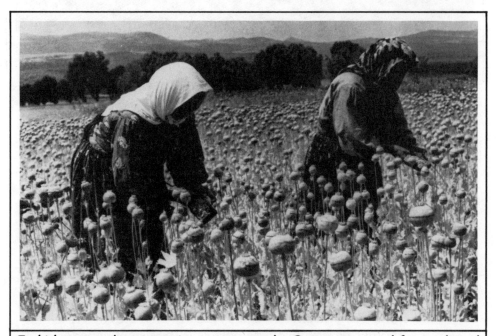

Turkish women harvest opium poppy seeds. Opium was used for medicinal purposes in the Near East as early as the 4th century C.E.

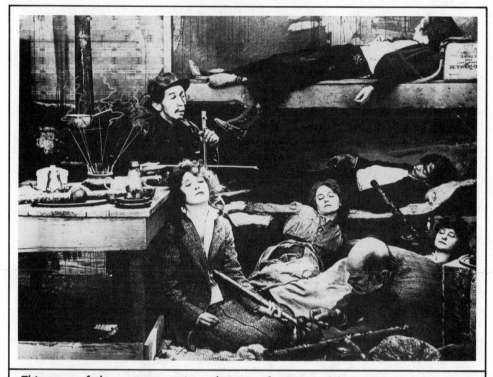

This turn-of-the-century opium den was frequented by working women. In the 1980s fewer women than men use heroin.

Opiates are powerful antitussive agents, which means that they prevent coughing. (Codeine is used in some cough medicines.) Nausea and vomiting can occur, especially on first contact with opiates. Actions on the skin include redness, itching, and sweating. "Pinpoint pupils" (or *miosis*) is another effect and is often used in diagnosing opiate overdose.

Death and Disease

As noted above, most deaths and other medical emergencies (such as coma) from overdose involve respiratory depression. Mixing heroin or other opiates with central nervous system depressants such as alcohol, barbiturates, or benzodiazepines (see Chapters 2 and 5) greatly increases this risk.

Another hazard involving opiates is the use of hypodermic needles to inject these drugs. Addicts often fail to sterilize their needles, or they share contaminated needles with fellow users. Infected or shared needles can easily transmit fatal diseases such as hepatitis and *acquired immune deficiency syndrome* (AIDS). One recent study found that more than 50% of intravenous heroin users were infected with the *human immunodeficiency virus* (HIV) responsible for AIDS. It has been suggested that this terrible disease may become the leading cause of death among intravenous drug abusers.

Women and Opiates

The effects of the opiates on women primarily involve problems in reproduction and the effects on the fetus and are dealt with in Chapter 8. It is important to note that many pain relievers (Demerol and codeine, for example) frequently prescribed for female patients are opiates. While not as powerful as morphine and heroin, heavy or long-term use of these drugs can lead to addiction or overdose.

NIDA figures for high-school seniors in the class of 1984 indicate that heroin use among students is low — only 1.0% of all women had ever tried it (compared with 1.5% of male students). The main problem with heroin use, apart from the medical hazards outlined above, is that it is strongly addictive. The financial strain of acquiring the drug, often on a daily basis for confirmed addicts, is constant. As in the case of some female cocaine addicts (see Chapter 4), many women must turn to prostitution to support their opiate habits. This can, of course, lead to further problems of venereal disease, unwanted pregnancies, emotional and economic degradation, and AIDS.

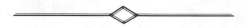

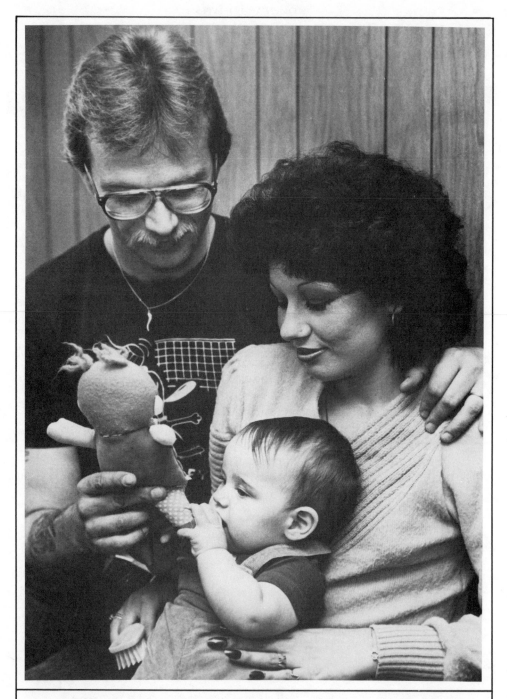

Two reformed heroin addicts with their baby. Women who use opiates while pregnant have a 60% to 90% chance of bearing an addicted child.

CHAPTER 8

DRUGS AND REPRODUCTION

During the nine months of pregnancy the expectant mother can do an enormous amount of good — or harm — to her child. As the fertilized egg develops into an embryo and then a fetus, the unborn child is dependent on the mother for oxygen, essential nutrients, protection, and removal of waste products. During this period of gestation, almost any substance — whether eaten, inhaled, or injected — entering the mother's bloodstream can also enter the fetal blood circulation and affect the development of the fetus. Psychoactive drugs such as those discussed in earlier chapters can have especially damaging effects on the developing fetus.

The effects of drug use during pregnancy is an enormous and complicated subject involving the evaluation of many drugs, ranging from aspirin and caffeine through alcohol and tobacco to illicit drugs such as cocaine and heroin. This chapter covers only the most important psychoactive drugs and is not intended as a complete guide to safe drug use during pregnancy. Any reader who is or might possibly be pregnant is urged immediately to consult a physician and other, more detailed sources of information. Needless to say, it can be difficult to talk about sensitive drug matters with doctors and other adults, but remember that in this case the results of drug use can affect not only the primary user, the woman, but can also permanently damage the fetus.

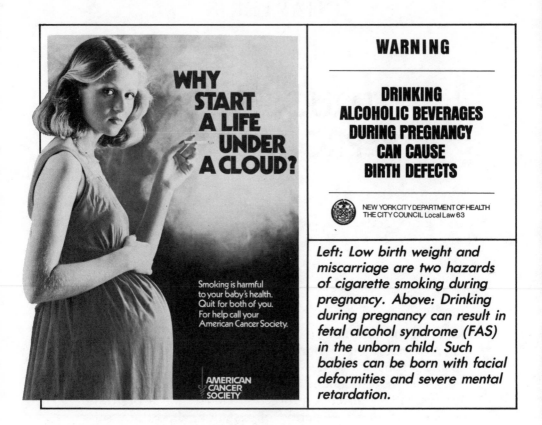

WARNING

DRINKING ALCOHOLIC BEVERAGES DURING PREGNANCY CAN CAUSE BIRTH DEFECTS

NEW YORK CITY DEPARTMENT OF HEALTH
THE CITY COUNCIL Local Law 63

Left: Low birth weight and miscarriage are two hazards of cigarette smoking during pregnancy. Above: Drinking during pregnancy can result in fetal alcohol syndrome (FAS) in the unborn child. Such babies can be born with facial deformities and severe mental retardation.

How Drugs Can Affect the Fetus

Any psychoactive substance — whether eaten, inhaled or injected — eventually reaches the user's bloodstream and enters the brain, where it exerts its mood-altering and other central nervous system effects. While in the bloodstream, these same substances can act on other organs and tissues to cause a variety of side effects, usually undesirable — in the skin, the liver, the heart, the intestines, and elsewhere throughout the body.

During pregnancy, the blood of the developing fetus is linked to the maternal bloodstream by a complex and vital organ, the placenta. In the placenta, blood traveling in the fetal circulatory system comes repeatedly into very close contact with that in the maternal circulatory system. This contact allows oxygen, vitamins, and other essential nutrients to pass from the mother to the fetus. At the same time, carbon dioxide and other waste products (such as those normally excreted in the urine in children and adults) pass from the fetus into the maternal bloodstream.

It was once thought that the placenta acted as a protective device to shield the fetus from harmful substances. It is now known, however, that many drugs — because of their small size, chemical structure, or similarity to natural biological molecules — cross the placenta and affect the fetal brain and organs as well as the mother. Drugs taken by the mother can be particularly harmful to the fetus since doses considered "normal" or "mild" for the mother are relatively much stronger and more toxic to the smaller fetus. In addition, the blood-brain barrier (a membrane separating the brain from the bloodstream that prevents some substances from reaching the brain) and organs such as the liver, which limit or regulate drug activity in humans, are not fully functioning in humans before birth. Especially severe damage can result from drug use early in pregnancy when the fetal brain, vital organs, and limbs develop. Virtually any drug, legal or illegal, can affect the fetus. Drug use of any kind during pregnancy should first be approved by a physician.

Fetal Alcohol Syndrome

Alcohol is a poison to the fetus just as it is to children and adults. In fact, maternal alcohol use during pregnancy is the third leading cause of mental retardation in children. Heavy or even moderate drinking by the mother can cause *fetal alcohol syndrome* (FAS), a severe and crippling affliction, in her offspring.

The greatest danger of maternal alcohol use is on the developing fetal nervous system. Babies with FAS demonstrate significantly low IQs and can be severely mentally retarded. *Microcephaly*, or small brain size, is another feature of babies suffering from FAS. Other problems involve characteristic facial deformities, slow growth and development, low birth weight, and a weakened immune system, leading to a more disease-prone child.

In addition, alcohol consumption during pregnancy can lead to miscarriage. One study indicated that pregnant women who have more than three drinks per day are two to three times more likely to suffer miscarriage or stillbirth than those having less than one drink per day. Newborn babies whose mothers drank during pregnancy can also display sleep disturbances and a weak sucking reflex. For the sake of the fetus, all alcoholic beverages should be avoided during pregnancy.

Tobacco and Fetal Toxins

When a pregnant woman smokes a cigarette, all the poisonous substances contained in tobacco cross the placenta and can damage the fetus. Just as with alcohol, scientists have conducted many studies concerning the dangers of using tobacco during pregnancy, and many hazards to the fetus have been conclusively identified.

One of the major fetal toxins in cigarette smoke is carbon monoxide. As described in Chapter 3, carbon monoxide reduces oxygen delivery in the blood and causes hypoxia, which in turn causes serious problems in the developing tissues and organs of the fetus. The nicotine contained in tobacco is a stimulant to the fetus, increasing the heart rate and further affecting oxygen circulation. Carcinogens such as benzopyrene may lead to increased cancer risks later in life.

Other possible dangers of cigarette smoking during pregnancy include miscarriage, premature birth, and greater risk of *sudden infant death syndrome* (the sudden death of a baby from an often unidentified cause). Significantly decreased birth weight is also well documented among offspring of mothers who smoke. Children of smokers are also much more likely to become smokers themselves.

Opiates

Unsurprisingly for such potent drugs, the use of opiates such as heroin and morphine during pregnancy causes serious problems for the fetus. These problems arise directly from the effects of the drug as well as from the opiate addict's lifestyle.

As with other drugs used during pregnancy, opiates increase the risk of miscarriage to almost twice the normal rate. Excessive bleeding during delivery, breech births, and stillbirths are also more common among maternal opiate users.

The babies born to these women are in effect addicted to opiates themselves and suffer from terrible withdrawal symptoms after birth. Neonatal withdrawal symptoms from heroin or morphine include high-pitched crying, irritability, sweating, mental disturbance and convulsions, sleeplessness, vomiting, and diarrhea. These can be serious medical emergencies in the newborn.

The respiratory depression caused by opiates in adults also affects the fetus and the newborn child. Pneumonia, *tachypnea* (rapid breathing), and other forms of respiratory distress are all common in babies born to opiate users.

Indirect problems related to opiate use include poor maternal (and thus fetal) nutrition, polydrug abuse, poor health care, and the serious risks of prenatal infection of AIDS, venereal disease, or other infections transmitted through needles or prostitution.

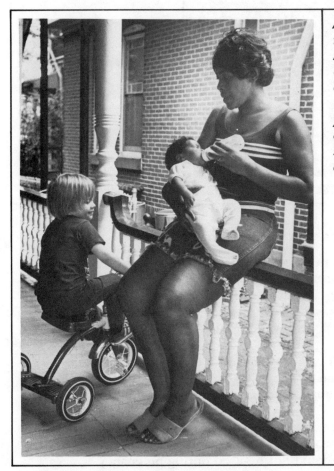

A former heroin addict feeds her infant. Approximately 9,000 children are born addicted to heroin in the United States every year. If left untreated, a newborn's withdrawal symptoms can be severe enough to cause death.

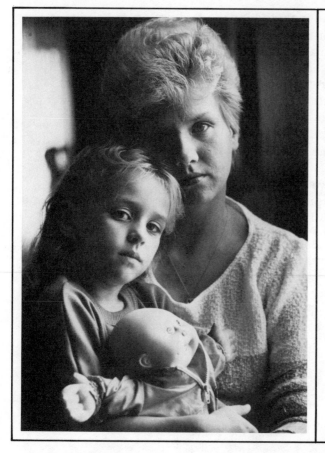

A mother with acquired immune deficiency syndrome (AIDS) and her healthy daughter. This tragic disease is prevalent among intravenous drug users and can be transmitted through contaminated hypodermic needles. During pregnancy an afflicted mother can transmit AIDS to her unborn child.

Cocaine and the Benzodiazepines

The recent epidemic of cocaine use in the form of crack has led to increased fears about the drug's effects during pregnancy. Babies born addicted to cocaine show signs of neurological disorder such as irritability, tremor, and muscle stiffness. Low birth weight, poor sucking, and diarrhea can also be present.

Maternal use during pregnancy of common tranquilizers (such as Valium and Librium) has been linked with increased risk of congenital malformations (birth defects) in the newborn. Some studies show that babies born to heavy benzodiazepine users are more likely to have cleft lip and palate and similar abnormalities. As with many prescription drugs, benzodiazepines should not be used during pregnancy.

Other Effects of Maternal Drug Use

As mentioned in reference to maternal opiate use, the use of drugs during pregnancy can affect the fetus and the newborn baby in indirect, nonpharmacological ways. Many drug users suffer from poverty, poor nutrition, lack of parental support, and poor health care. Financial hardship or lack of emotional support can lead to other problems, both before and after childbirth. In some cases, the stress and emotional upset associated with pregnancy can incite the expectant mother to further drug use, particularly of alcohol.

Most tragically, perhaps, maternal and fetal drug problems can prevent the crucial emotional bonding between mother and infant during the first few days of life — bonding that is vital to the development of a happy, healthy, and well-adjusted child.

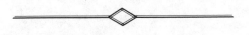

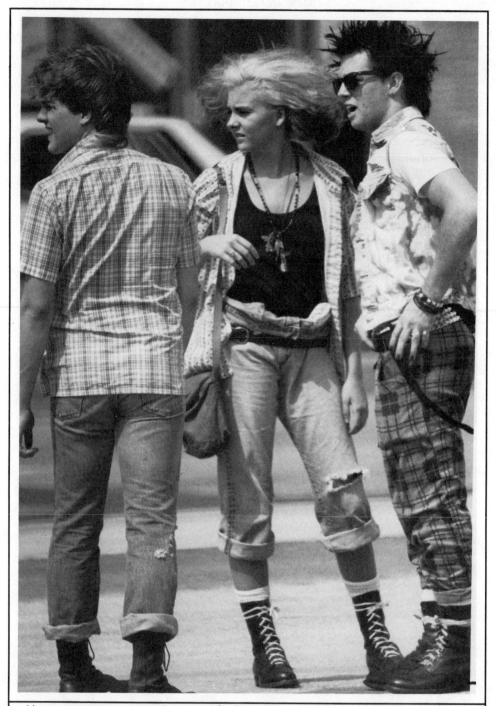

Many teenagers experiment with drugs in a quest for social acceptance. The consequences, including long-term addiction, can be disastrous.

CHAPTER 9

A NOTE TO TEENAGE READERS

High-school girls and other young women reading this book may understandably feel that much of its contents has little to do with them and their daily lives. The problems of employment, marriage, families, and pregnancy can seem distant and of little importance to teenagers more interested in juggling the demands of school and social life and caught up in the emotional turmoil of adolescence.

Use of psychoactive drugs, however, is certainly a concern among young people and, as this book shows, presents special problems for women of all ages. For teenagers, drugs can seriously interfere with school, social life, and family relations, as well as causing the various health problems covered in previous chapters. Young women must be especially concerned with unwanted pregnancies, permanent damage to their reproductive system, and other hazards, such as infectious disease and prostitution, linked to drug use by women.

Much of the content of earlier chapters involves fairly sophisticated scientific and medical terminology and concepts. Although it is included to aid in understanding how psychoactive drugs work (and possibly to awaken an interest in psychopharmacology), it is more important for teenagers simply to remember the few essential features and hazards of these common substances.

Alcohol use is widespread and socially accepted, which adds to its natural addictive potential. As well as long-term damage to the brain, liver, heart, and other organs, acute dangers include death from overdose and, more commonly, from automobile accidents. Mixing other drugs, especially depressants, with alcohol is extremely dangerous. Alcohol use by women can lead to inappropriate sexual activity and pregnancy. Alcohol severely damages the fetus and should not be used at all during pregnancy.

The tobacco contained in cigarettes contains many hazardous substances, most notably nicotine, carbon monoxide, and tar. These have all been linked to a number of severe diseases such as heart and lung disease and cancer. Nicotine is very addictive; a few cigarettes "now and then" can lead quickly to a pack-a-day habit. In women, tobacco damages the reproductive system and increases the dangers of the birth control pill. Cigarette smoking endangers pregnancy and harms the fetus. The easiest way to quit smoking seems to be "cold turkey," or in other words, by stopping abruptly.

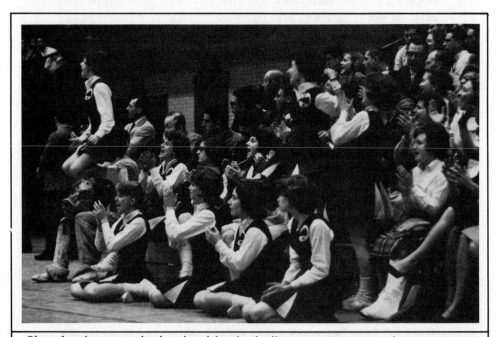

Cheerleaders at a high school basketball game. Sports and exercise are a healthy alternative to drugs for all teenagers.

Because teenage pregnancy is becoming a national problem, it is necessary for both schools and parents to educate young people about the consequences of sexual activity.

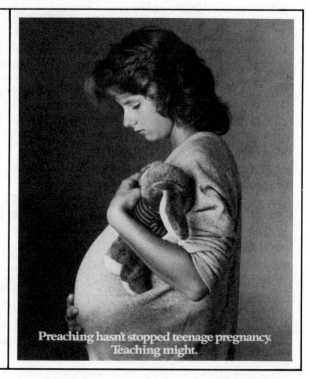

Preaching hasn't stopped teenage pregnancy. Teaching might.

Stimulant drugs such as amphetamines and cocaine are also addictive. Effects on the heart and blood vessels can cause immediate death. Long-term use leads to profound psychological changes such as paranoia and psychosis. Attempted weight loss through amphetamine use is temporary and dangerous and can lead to addiction. Because of its extreme addictiveness and high price, cocaine can induce women to turn to prostitution to pay for their habit.

Central nervous system depressants include barbiturates and tranquilizers such as Valium. These also are addictive, and tolerance soon develops so that higher doses are required for the same effect. All depressants are extremely dangerous in high doses and when mixed with alcohol. Mental processes and skills such as driving are also affected. Doctors often prescribe minor tranquilizers, usually benzodiazepines, to women because these drugs can reduce anxiety and sleeplessness. Such drugs should be used in low doses and for short-term therapy only. Barbiturates significantly decrease the effectiveness of the birth control pill. Both barbiturates

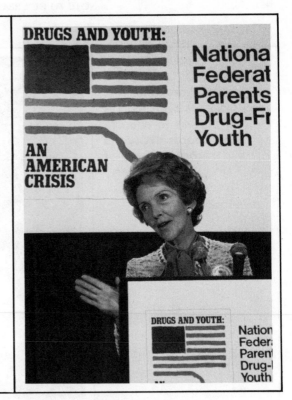

First Lady Nancy Reagan addresses a 1982 conference of the National Federation of Parents for Drug-Free Youth. Both Mrs. Reagan and the panel believe that educating young people about the effects of psychoactive substances is an essential part of the battle against drug abuse.

and tranquilizers can damage the fetus and should not be used during pregnancy.

Heroin and morphine are the most commonly abused opiates, although codeine and other painkillers belong to the same drug family. Hazards include death from overdose, other poisons mixed with the drug by dealers, and a variety of serious effects throughout the body. Intravenous injection of these or any drugs can transmit the deadly AIDS virus, which is increasingly a major cause of death among intravenous drug users. Heroin and other opiate addictions among women often lead to prostitution and further risks of AIDS, venereal disease, and unwanted pregnancy. Opiate use during pregnancy can damage or kill the fetus or lead to the birth of a baby already addicted to the drug.

Marijuana, hashish, and other cannabinoids are psychologically addicting and can cause drowsiness, memory problems, apathy, compulsive drug seeking, and other symptoms of the cannabinoid amotivational syndrome. This can cause obvious problems with schoolwork and jobs. In addition, studies show that marijuana use has been associated with experimentation with other drugs. Long-term heavy use can severely damage the lungs and other organs.

All young women should acquaint themselves with how their reproductive system functions. Simple understanding of the menstrual cycle, pregnancy, and methods of contraception is essential knowledge for any young woman but particularly for one who is using alcohol, cigarettes, or other psychoactive substances. Most important, pregnant women should consult a physician immediately to learn how to bear a happy, healthy child free from the damage of maternal drug abuse. If confidentiality is a concern, telephone "hot lines" or advisory services are available in many areas for initial consultation and advice.

In general, it is a good idea to understand the reasons for and the nature of any prescription medicine taken and to be aware of proper dosage and of how long the pills should be taken. It is important to realize that some of the painkillers prescribed for common problems such as recurring backache and menstrual cramps contain potentially addictive substances such as codeine. Most libraries contain at least one general, nontechnical guide to prescription drugs, and such a volume is a useful addition to any household bookshelf. Because of individual variation (such as allergies or liver problems), nearly any drug, and certainly those such as tranquilizers, can cause a variety of side effects in a user, some of which can be quite serious and even fatal. Anyone experiencing unexpected side effects from a drug should contact a physician immediately.

Most drugs offer a brief — and at times very welcome — high and a temporary escape from the stresses and difficulties of school, family life, emotional problems, and social pressures. Unfortunately, once the high wears off the hazards of drug use remain: overdose and death, long-term damage to the body and mind, addiction and relentless craving for a drug, academic failure, further emotional problems, and, for a woman, the many special dangers involving her complex and fragile reproductive system.

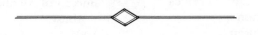

APPENDIX

State Agencies for the Prevention and Treatment of Drug Abuse

ALABAMA
Department of Mental Health
Division of Mental Illness and
  Substance Abuse Community
  Programs
200 Interstate Park Drive
P.O. Box 3710
Montgomery, AL 36193
(205) 271-9253

ALASKA
Department of Health and Social
  Services
Office of Alcoholism and Drug
  Abuse
Pouch H-05-F
Juneau, AK 99811
(907) 586-6201

ARIZONA
Department of Health Services
Division of Behavioral Health
  Services
Bureau of Community Services
Alcohol Abuse and Alcoholism
  Section
2500 East Van Buren
Phoenix, AZ 85008
(602) 255-1238

Department of Health Services
Division of Behavioral Health
  Services
Bureau of Community Services
Drug Abuse Section
2500 East Van Buren
Phoenix, AZ 85008
(602) 255-1240

ARKANSAS
Department of Human Services
Office on Alcohol and Drug Abuse
  Prevention
1515 West 7th Avenue
Suite 310
Little Rock, AR 72202
(501) 371-2603

CALIFORNIA
Department of Alcohol and Drug
  Abuse
111 Capitol Mall
Sacramento, CA 95814
(916) 445-1940

COLORADO
Department of Health
Alcohol and Drug Abuse Division
4210 East 11th Avenue
Denver, CO 80220
(303) 320-6137

CONNECTICUT
Alcohol and Drug Abuse
  Commission
999 Asylum Avenue
3rd Floor
Hartford, CT 06105
(203) 566-4145

DELAWARE
Division of Mental Health
Bureau of Alcoholism and Drug
  Abuse
1901 North Dupont Highway
Newcastle, DE 19720
(302) 421-6101

DISTRICT OF COLUMBIA
Department of Human Services
Office of Health Planning and
  Development
601 Indiana Avenue, NW
Suite 500
Washington, D.C. 20004
(202) 724-5641

FLORIDA
Department of Health and
  Rehabilitative Services
Alcoholic Rehabilitation Program
1317 Winewood Boulevard
Room 187A
Tallahassee, FL 32301
(904) 488-0396

Department of Health and
  Rehabilitative Services
Drug Abuse Program
1317 Winewood Boulevard
Building 6, Room 155
Tallahassee, FL 32301
(904) 488-0900

GEORGIA
Department of Human Resources
Division of Mental Health and
  Mental Retardation
Alcohol and Drug Section
618 Ponce De Leon Avenue, NE
Atlanta, GA 30365-2101
(404) 894-4785

HAWAII
Department of Health
Mental Health Division
Alcohol and Drug Abuse Branch
1250 Punch Bowl Street
P.O. Box 3378
Honolulu, HI 96801
(808) 548-4280

IDAHO
Department of Health and Welfare
Bureau of Preventive Medicine
Substance Abuse Section
450 West State
Boise, ID 83720
(208) 334-4368

ILLINOIS
Department of Mental Health and
  Developmental Disabilities
Division of Alcoholism
160 North La Salle Street
Room 1500
Chicago, IL 60601
(312) 793-2907

Illinois Dangerous Drugs
  Commission
300 North State Street
Suite 1500
Chicago, IL 60610
(312) 822-9860

INDIANA
Department of Mental Health
Division of Addiction Services
429 North Pennsylvania Street
Indianapolis, IN 46204
(317) 232-7816

IOWA
Department of Substance Abuse
505 5th Avenue
Insurance Exchange Building
Suite 202
Des Moines, IA 50319
(515) 281-3641

KANSAS
Department of Social Rehabilitation
Alcohol and Drug Abuse Services
2700 West 6th Street
Biddle Building
Topeka, KS 66606
(913) 296-3925

KENTUCKY
Cabinet for Human Resources
Department of Health Services
Substance Abuse Branch
275 East Main Street
Frankfort, KY 40601
(502) 564-2880

LOUISIANA
Department of Health and Human
  Resources
Office of Mental Health and
  Substance Abuse
655 North 5th Street
P.O. Box 4049
Baton Rouge, LA 70821
(504) 342-2565

MAINE
Department of Human Services
Office of Alcoholism and Drug
  Abuse Prevention
Bureau of Rehabilitation
32 Winthrop Street
Augusta, ME 04330
(207) 289-2781

MARYLAND
Alcoholism Control Administration
201 West Preston Street
Fourth Floor
Baltimore, MD 21201
(301) 383-2977

State Health Department
Drug Abuse Administration
201 West Preston Street
Baltimore, MD 21201
(301) 383-3312

MASSACHUSETTS
Department of Public Health
Division of Alcoholism
755 Boylston Street
Sixth Floor
Boston, MA 02116
(617) 727-1960

Department of Public Health
Division of Drug Rehabilitation
600 Washington Street
Boston, MA 02114
(617) 727-8617

MICHIGAN
Department of Public Health
Office of Substance Abuse Services
3500 North Logan Street
P.O. Box 30035
Lansing, MI 48909
(517) 373-8603

MINNESOTA
Department of Public Welfare
Chemical Dependency Program
  Division
Centennial Building
658 Cedar Street
4th Floor
Saint Paul, MN 55155
(612) 296-4614

MISSISSIPPI
Department of Mental Health
Division of Alcohol and Drug Abuse
1102 Robert E. Lee Building
Jackson, MS 39201
(601) 359-1297

MISSOURI
Department of Mental Health
Division of Alcoholism and Drug
  Abuse
2002 Missouri Boulevard
P.O. Box 687
Jefferson City, MO 65102
(314) 751-4942

MONTANA
Department of Institutions
Alcohol and Drug Abuse Division
1539 11th Avenue
Helena, MT 59620
(406) 449-2827

NEBRASKA
Department of Public Institutions
Division of Alcoholism and Drug Abuse
801 West Van Dorn Street
P.O. Box 94728
Lincoln, NB 68509
(402) 471-2851, Ext. 415

NEVADA
Department of Human Resources
Bureau of Alcohol and Drug Abuse
505 East King Street
Carson City, NV 89710
(702) 885-4790

NEW HAMPSHIRE
Department of Health and Welfare
Office of Alcohol and Drug Abuse
   Prevention
Hazen Drive
Health and Welfare Building
Concord, NH 03301
(603) 271-4627

NEW JERSEY
Department of Health
Division of Alcoholism
129 East Hanover Street CN 362
Trenton, NJ 08625
(609) 292-8949

Department of Health
Division of Narcotic and Drug Abuse
   Control
129 East Hanover Street CN 362
Trenton, NJ 08625
(609) 292-8949

NEW MEXICO
Health and Environment Department
Behavioral Services Division
Substance Abuse Bureau
725 Saint Michaels Drive
P.O. Box 968
Santa Fe, NM 87503
(505) 984-0020, Ext. 304

NEW YORK
Division of Alcoholism and Alcohol
   Abuse
194 Washington Avenue
Albany, NY 12210
(518) 474-5417

Division of Substance Abuse
   Services
Executive Park South
Box 8200
Albany, NY 12203
(518) 457-7629

NORTH CAROLINA
Department of Human Resources
Division of Mental Health, Mental
   Retardation and Substance Abuse
   Services
Alcohol and Drug Abuse Services
325 North Salisbury Street
Albemarle Building
Raleigh, NC 27611
(919) 733-4670

NORTH DAKOTA
Department of Human Services
Division of Alcoholism and Drug
   Abuse
State Capitol Building
Bismarck, ND 58505
(701) 224-2767

OHIO
Department of Health
Division of Alcoholism
246 North High Street
P.O. Box 118
Columbus, OH 43216
(614) 466-3543

Department of Mental Health
Bureau of Drug Abuse
65 South Front Street
Columbus, OH 43215
(614) 466-9023

OKLAHOMA
Department of Mental Health
Alcohol and Drug Programs
4545 North Lincoln Boulevard
Suite 100 East Terrace
P.O. Box 53277
Oklahoma City, OK 73152
(405) 521-0044

OREGON
Department of Human Resources
Mental Health Division
Office of Programs for Alcohol and
  Drug Problems
2575 Bittern Street, NE
Salem, OR 97310
(503) 378-2163

PENNSYLVANIA
Department of Health
Office of Drug and Alcohol
  Programs
Commonwealth and Forster Avenues
Health and Welfare Building
P.O. Box 90
Harrisburg, PA 17108
(717) 787-9857

RHODE ISLAND
Department of Mental Health,
  Mental Retardation and Hospitals
Division of Substance Abuse
Substance Abuse Administration
  Building
Cranston, RI 02920
(401) 464-2091

SOUTH CAROLINA
Commission on Alcohol and Drug
  Abuse
3700 Forest Drive
Columbia, SC 29204
(803) 758-2521

SOUTH DAKOTA
Department of Health
Division of Alcohol and Drug Abuse
523 East Capitol, Joe Foss Building
Pierre, SD 57501
(605) 773-4806

TENNESSEE
Department of Mental Health and
  Mental Retardation
Alcohol and Drug Abuse Services
505 Deaderick Street
James K. Polk Building, Fourth Floor
Nashville, TN 37219
(615) 741-1921

TEXAS
Commission on Alcoholism
809 Sam Houston State Office Building
Austin, TX 78701
(512) 475-2577

Department of Community Affairs
Drug Abuse Prevention Division
2015 South Interstate Highway 35
P.O. Box 13166
Austin, TX 78711
(512) 443-4100

UTAH
Department of Social Services
Division of Alcoholism and Drugs
150 West North Temple
Suite 350
P.O. Box 2500
Salt Lake City, UT 84110
(801) 533-6532

VERMONT
Agency of Human Services
Department of Social and
  Rehabilitation Services
Alcohol and Drug Abuse Division
103 South Main Street
Waterbury, VT 05676
(802) 241-2170

VIRGINIA

Department of Mental Health and
Mental Retardation
Division of Substance Abuse
109 Governor Street
P.O. Box 1797
Richmond, VA 23214
(804) 786-5313

WASHINGTON

Department of Social and Health
Service
Bureau of Alcohol and Substance
Abuse
Office Building—44 W
Olympia, WA 98504
(206) 753-5866

WEST VIRGINIA

Department of Health
Office of Behavioral Health Services
Division on Alcoholism and Drug
Abuse
1800 Washington Street East
Building 3 Room 451
Charleston, WV 25305
(304) 348-2276

WISCONSIN

Department of Health and Social
Services
Division of Community Services
Bureau of Community Programs
Alcohol and Other Drug Abuse
Program Office
1 West Wilson Street
P.O. Box 7851
Madison, WI 53707
(608) 266-2717

WYOMING

Alcohol and Drug Abuse Programs
Hathaway Building
Cheyenne, WY 82002
(307) 777-7115, Ext. 7118

GUAM

Mental Health & Substance Abuse
Agency
P.O. Box 20999
Guam 96921

PUERTO RICO

Department of Addiction Control
Services
Alcohol Abuse Programs
P.O. Box B-Y Rio Piedras Station
Rio Piedras, PR 00928
(809) 763-5014

Department of Addiction Control
Services
Drug Abuse Programs
P.O. Box B-Y Rio Piedras Station
Rio Piedras, PR 00928
(809) 764-8140

VIRGIN ISLANDS

Division of Mental Health,
Alcoholism & Drug Dependency
Services
P.O. Box 7329
Saint Thomas, Virgin Islands 00801
(809) 774-7265

AMERICAN SAMOA

LBJ Tropical Medical Center
Department of Mental Health Clinic
Pago Pago, American Samoa 96799

TRUST TERRITORIES

Director of Health Services
Office of the High Commissioner
Saipan, Trust Territories 96950

FURTHER READING

Alibrandi, Tom. *Young Alcoholics*. Minneapolis: CompCare Publications, 1978.

Corrigan, Eileen M. *Alcoholic Women in Treatment*. New York: Oxford University Press, 1980.

Gordon, Barbara. *I'm Dancing As Fast As I Can*. New York: Harper & Row, 1979.

Harkness, Richard. *Drug Interactions Handbook*. Englewood Cliffs, New Jersey: Prentice-Hall, 1984.

Jones-Witters, Patricia and Witters, Weldon. *Drugs and Society: A Biological Perspective*. Monterey, California: Wadsworth Health Sciences, 1983.

Nellis, Muriel. *The Female Fix*. New York: Houghton Mifflin, 1980.

Stimel, Barry. *The Effects of Maternal Alcohol and Drug Abuse on the Newborn*. New York: Haworth Press, 1982.

GLOSSARY

acetylcholine a neurotransmitter that plays an important role in the transmission of nerve impulses, especially at synapses. Nicotine mimics its action at nicotinic receptors

acquired immune deficiency syndrome a fatal disease caused by the human immunodeficiency virus; it is transmitted via sexual contact and by intravenous injection of drugs or blood transfusion; also known as AIDS

addiction a condition caused by repeated drug use, characterized by a compulsive urge to continue using the drug, a tendency to increase the dosage, and physiological and/or psychological dependence

adrenalin a hormone that the body releases in times of stress; also referred to as epinephrine

anorectic having no appetite

anovular cycle a menstrual cycle in which ovulation does not occur before the menstrual flow

antiemetic a drug that prevents vomiting, often by actions on a specific portion of the brain known as the chemoreceptor trigger zone

antitussives drugs that reduce coughing

anxiolytics drugs such as tranquilizers that reduce feelings of anxiety

atherosclerosis a disease wherein fatty deposits grow on the inner walls of arteries and eventually interfere with normal blood flow

autonomic nervous system the part of the nervous system concerned with control of involuntary bodily functions

benzodiazepines a family of tranquilizers — including Valium and Librium—used medically for their mildly sedating effects

benzopyrene an important carcinogen present in tobacco tar

blood-brain barrier a semipermeable membrane that separates circulating blood from tissue fluid surrounding brain cells, thus protecting the brain from some poisons and buildup of unwanted chemicals

bronchitis damage to the respiratory pathways leading to heavy coughing and difficulty in breathing

cannabinoids psychoactive chemicals found in marijuana

carcinogen a substance that causes cancer

cardiac arrythmias irregular heart rhythms, sometimes accompanied by symptoms such as palpitations, breathlessness and chest pains. In serious cases, this condition can lead to cardiac arrest

cardiomyopathy any chronic problem that, in turn, damages the muscles of the heart

cardiovascular relating to the heart and blood vessels

central nervous system consisting of the brain, spinal cord and connecting nerves, which together control the body's voluntary acts

cerebrovascular relating to the blood vessels of the brain

chemoreceptor trigger zone a region of the brain which, when stimulated, can cause vomiting; site of many antiemetics

cirrhosis a chronic, deteriorating disease of the liver

coma profound unconsciousness where the patient does not respond to external stimuli. More than half the number of victims that suffer comas were initially afflicted by a trauma to the head or brain occurring as a result of accident or injury

conjunctiva the delicate mucous membrane lining the inner portion of the eyelids

coping mechanism psychological term referring to an individual's methods of handling a challenge

detoxification the body's process for removing poisonous substances or rendering them harmless. The liver often performs this function

emphysema severe destruction of lung tissue, leading to extreme difficulty in breathing

encephalopathy a general medical term denoting various diseases that can damage the brain

endogenous referring to a natural substance produced by the body

GABA receptors receptors for the important inhibitory neurotransmitter gamma-aminobutyric acid, found in the central nervous system and brain. Benzodiazepines such as Valium affect GABA receptors

ganglion junctions within the nervous system between two neurons; sites where neurotransmitters act on receptors

gestation the period of time that begins with the fertilization of an ovum by a sperm and continues to childbirth

hemoglobin a protein in red blood cells carrying oxygen from the lungs to body tissues

hypothalamus a frontal region of the brain containing several neurosecretions that regulate body temperature, appetite, thirst, and sexual behavior

hypoxia a condition where the body's tissues are deprived of oxygen

immune system the body's system of protection against infection and disease, based mainly on specialized cells and proteins (called antibodies) circulating in the bloodstream. The AIDS virus kills by rendering this system ineffective

insomnia a state of sleeplessness, often caused by anxiety or depression

metabolites substances produced by internal chemical reactions or obtained from injected food matter, which play a part in metabolic processes of the body

miosis constriction of the pupils, occurring in severe form as a result of opiate use

narcotics drugs that produce sleep and relieve pain in small doses, but produce unconsciousness and stupors in larger amounts; examples of these drugs are opium, codeine, morphine and heroin

neuron the individual structural units that, when linked together, comprise the nervous system and act to initiate and conduct impulses throughout the body; neurons are also called nerve cells

neurotransmitter the chemical substances that one neuron releases to transmit impulses to the receptors of other neurons. Many psychoactive drugs work on the body by mimicking, preventing, prolonging or enhancing the actions of certain neurotransmitters

nicotinic receptor receptors located throughout the body that are stimulated by both acetylcholine and nicotine

noradrenaline a hormone chemically related to adrenaline that causes many similar body reactions when secreted, such as an increase in blood pressure and an accelerated breathing rate; also known as norepinephrine

opiates compounds derived from the milky juice of the poppy plant *Papaver somniferum*, including opium, morphine, codeine and their derivatives, such as heroin

opioids natural or endogenous chemicals that have pain-relieving properties, including endorphins, enkephalins and dynorphins. Opiates work by mimicking these natural substances

physical dependence adaption of the body to the presence of a drug such that its absence produces withdrawal symptoms

placenta an organ which mediates transfer of oxygen, nutrients and waste products between mother and fetus

prostacyclin one of an important family of fatty acid derivatives known as prostaglandins. Prostacyclin works to maintain blood fluidity and reduce unnecessary clotting

psychological dependence a condition in which the drug user craves a drug to maintain a sense of well-being and feels discomfort when deprived of it

psychosis severe mental derangement where a patient abnormally perceives reality and experiences severe personality changes

receptor a specialized component of a cell that combines with a chemical substance to trigger an impulse in the cell; for example, nerve cell receptors combine with neurotransmitters

respiratory center that part of the brain controlling respiratory function

respiratory depression reduced breathing and possible widespread hypoxia caused by damage to or poisoning of the respiratory center

reuptake the removal of excess neurotransmitters from the synaptic region back into the neuron that released them

stroke weakness or paralysis affecting certain regions of the body and occasionally accompanied by damage to the brain. This condition is caused most commonly by an interruption in the normal flow of blood to the brain

sympathetic nervous system a division of the autonomic nervous system that regulates such activities as hormone secretion and heartbeat

tolerance a decrease of susceptibility to the effects of a drug due to its continued administration, resulting in the user's need to increase the drug dosage in order to achieve the desired effects

tranquilizers drugs that act to produce calming effects and relieve anxiety, while not interfering with normal mental activities. Some of these tranquilizers, commonly known by their trade names, are Librium, Thorazine, Valium, Miltown, Sparine, and Serpasil

withdrawal the physiological and psychological effects of discontinued use of a drug

PICTURE CREDITS

American Cancer Society: pp. 44, 52; B. Anspach/Art Resource: pp. 10, 36; AP/Wide World Photos: pp. 32, 70, 71, 76, 78, 82, 88, 94; Art Resource: pp. 64, 68; The Bettmann Archive: pp. 22, 28, 34, 46, 50; Bildarchiv Foto Marburg/Art Resource: p. 31; A. Chwatsky/Art Resource: p. 25; J. Gill/Art Resource: p. 39; E. Luttenberg/Art Resource: P. 62; National Library of Medicine: p. 79; Planned Parenthood: pp. 42, 99; A Sidorfsky/Art Resource: p. 18; Snark/Art Resource: p. 12; United Nations: p. 33; UPI/Bettmann Newsphotos: pp. 26, 29, 41, 43, 54, 57, 58, 60, 67, 73, 80, 84, 85, 86, 93, 96, 98, 100

Original illustrations by Gary Tong: pp. 20, 48, 49, 51, 59, 72

Index

Paul Nordstrom August is a biotechnical and pharmaceutical writer whose expertise extends to such subjects as public health policies, medical politics, and psychopharmacology. He holds a B.A. in English literature from Stanford University and is a medical student at Guy's Hospital Medical School, London.

Solomon H. Snyder, M.D., is Distinguished Service Professor of Neuroscience, Pharmacology and Psychiatry at The Johns Hopkins University School of Medicine. He has served as president of the Society for Neuroscience and in 1978 received the Albert Lasker Award in Medical Research. He has authored *Uses of Marijuana, Madness and the Brain, The Troubled Mind, Biological Aspects of Mental Disorder,* and edited *Perspective in Neuropharmacology: A Tribute to Julius Axelrod.* Professor Snyder was a research associate with Dr. Axelrod at the National Institutes of Health.

Barry L. Jacobs, Ph.D., is currently a professor in the program of neuroscience at Princeton University. Professor Jacobs is author of *Serotonin Neurotransmission and Behavior* and *Hallucinogens: Neurochemical, Behavioral and Clinical Perspectives.* He has written many journal articles in the field of neuroscience and contributed numerous chapters to books on behavior and brain science. He has been a member of several panels of the National Institute of Mental Health.

Joann Ellison Rodgers, M.S. (Columbia), became Deputy Director of Public Affairs and Director of Media Relations for the Johns Hopkins Medical Institutions in Baltimore, Maryland, in 1984 after 18 years as an award-winning science journalist and widely read columnist for the Hearst newspapers.